Wellness in Menopause

A Guide to Holistic Healing

MARYLYN MEEK

Newleaf

Newleaf
an imprint of
Gill & Macmillan Ltd
Hume Avenue
Park West
Dublin 12
with associated companies throughout the world
www.gillmacmillan.ie

© *2000 Marylyn Meek*
0 7171 0064 2

Index compiled by Helen Litton
Design by Carole Lynch
Print origination by O'K Graphic Design, Dublin
Printed by ColourBooks Ltd, Dublin

A catalogue record is available for this book from
the British Library.

1 3 5 4 2

Contents

Acknowledgments

Montse Bradford (Macrobiotics) Greenfields, Lovington, Castle Cary, Somerset BA7 7PX.
Dietary counselling and cooking classes in Somerset and London. Write for details.
Celia Hewson BA, MIFA, ITEC, LL.SA (Hons) (Aromatherapy) Taunton, Somerset. Tel.: (01823) 252443.
Kristin Jeffs MCPP (Herbal Medicine)
Wells, Somerset. Tel.: (01749) 675352.
Andrew Johnson MH, DT, RIr. (Nutritional Therapy)
Associate Member of the Ayurvedic Medical Association UK.
East West Centre, 10 High Street, Glastonbury, Somerset BA6 9DU. Tel./fax: (01458) 833382.
Ms Li Li MBAcC (Traditional Chinese Medicine), Practitioner of Acupuncture and Chinese Medicine, Member of British Acupuncture Council.
Catherine Macleod (Counselling—Intuitive Guidance)
Write for details enclosing a sae to:
c/o 2 Lower Farm Cottages, Lottisham, Nr. Baltonsborough, Glastonbury, Somerset BA6 8PF.
Elizabeth Rugman ITEC, IHBC (Reflexology)
9 Straightmead, Litton, Chewton Mendip, Nr. Bath, BA3 4PW. Tel.: (01761) 241473.
Dr Lesley Strutte) MB. BS. DObst., RCOG, MF Hom. (Homoeopathy)
Langport, Somerset. Tel.: (01458) 850357.

With thanks also to: Alick Bartholomew, Tony Payne, Group Leader, Meditation Group, NFSH Healing Centre, Glastonbury for his help and guidance over the years; Mark Bishop for the information on Shiatsu; Celia Wright at Higher Nature for her willing assistance; Caroline Pickford for getting me off to a flying start with the typing; Laurence McLeod-Sharpe for his computer wizardry; to everyone at Newleaf for their faith and support—with special thanks to Tina Currie for her inspired editing. And special thanks to Catherine for her help and encouragement throughout and my son Rory for his forebearance and help at home.

Introduction

Observing that many women suffer needlessly during the menopausal phase of their lives prompted me to put together this simple guide. It looks at elected holistic therapies and their use in treating the specific ailments connected with this natural process.

The aim of this book is to help women understand and pass through the menopause in a positive way. I offer suggestions about making changes in lifestyle and attitudes as a means of restoring the body to its natural balance and harmony.

Readers are recommended to pay particular attention to any stated cautions in respect of self-treatment, although no recommended remedy included in this book can have harmful effects if the guidelines are followed. I hope you will find the self-help measures useful, but for further help a qualified practitioner should be consulted.

I am very grateful for the specialist help afforded to me by the therapists listed in the acknowledgements.

CHAPTER ONE

A Time of Change

When a woman is around the age of forty, various hormonal and glandular changes take place which mark the onset of her climacteric, or change of life. This heralds the beginning of a gradual decrease of the production in her body of two hormones, first oestrogen and then, when ovulation has ceased, progesterone.

This change, normally spanning fifteen to twenty years, has many recorded symptoms attributed to it. Although some women appear to encounter few difficulties and have little to complain about, many are less fortunate. A fairly high percentage suffer the familiar menopausal distress of hot flushes, depression, mood swings and tiredness. About eighty per cent of all women suffer some degree of symptoms during this phase of their lives.

The menopause is a major life passage occurring in the middle of this larger picture of winding down. A natural process, it can take anything from six months to three years to pass through. It most commonly occurs between the ages of forty-eight and fifty-two and marks the end of fertility and the menstrual cycle. Among the early signals that ovulation is no longer taking place are a lengthening or variation in the monthly menstrual cycle, a lack of energy and a greater emotional sensitivity.

Women's attitudes to the menopause have long been influenced and shaped by myth, culture and the conditioning of society. For many generations, the greater proportion of the world's female population has been under male domination. Women have largely been encouraged in the negative beliefs that their value, desirability and sexual fulfilment cease when they are no longer able to maintain their reproductive role. Until recently, the subject of sexuality in our society has been taboo. Lack of support and communication have created a sense of isolation, and it is not surprising that, for many women, this phase in their lives has been a source of fear and unhappiness.

During the latter half of this century, however, there has been a noticeable shift in women's attitude towards their sexuality. Combined with their more prominent role in the workplace has come evidence of their openly joining together to share problems and support each other. As they work side by side with men on a more equal footing than ever before, all the signs are that women are on the threshold of seeking a greater understanding of their personal power.

In many cultures, women traditionally have a positive view of letting go of those parts of their femininity which have been of service. They are encouraged to feel that they still retain their womanly value and to see the menopause as passing through a gateway to a new dimension of freedom, enhanced spirituality and wisdom. Women who adopt this attitude generally experience fewer symptoms.

With more information and help now filtering through from both conventional medical and alternative sources, women are realising that they *do* have more control in determining the type of passage they experience. The hormonal balance in the body is dependent on many factors—for instance, the way it is nourished both with food and quality of life. A correct diet suited to every woman's individual needs is of fundamental importance, coupled with a healthy lifestyle and regular exercise. Together, these act as building blocks, helping this time of potential transformation to be a rich and productive one.

CHAPTER TWO

The Natural Approach

The cure of the part should not be attempted without treatment of the whole.   Plato (428-348 BC)

HISTORICAL AND CURRENT TRENDS

We have come a long way from those ancient superstitious days when illness was thought to be caused by evil spirits or the wrath of the gods in response to the sinful behaviour of human beings. Even further back in history, there was a time when the human race was composed of simple, intuitive beings, in touch with their needs and able, like the animals, to recognise the plants and substances in their environment that possessed healing properties.

The almost meteoric growth in popularity of natural medicine, practices and disciplines in recent years is giving rise to a greater interest among people in the management of their own health and in the methods now available to them. Although some natural therapies are comparatively new, there are many—such as herbalism, Chinese medicine and the Ayurvedic system of India—which have traditionally been used for many thousands of years. In many other countries today, traditional practitioners and doctors of conventional medicine work side by side, respecting the benefits and advantages of each other's types of treatment. There are hopeful signs that this merging of scientific and holistic methods could one day evolve into an exciting third healthcare system.

Although the remarkable advances made by medicine since the beginning of the last century have undoubtedly saved countless lives and the system has a permanent place in society, there are clear signs of public dissatisfaction and a desire to consider alternatives. Orthodox medicine appears to have failed to:

(a) address the underlying causes of chronic or degenerative disease
(b) provide a source of lasting cure
(c) give the patient sufficient consultation time.

Increased public awareness of possible side-effects from drugs has also directed attention to natural methods.

The realisation of the need, in these stressful times, to talk about problems which could be affecting bodily health and the difficulty in which this places doctors has given rise to the practice of counselling and a move towards natural therapies, both ancient and modern. In holistic consultations, this type of discussion is treated as a relevant part of the practitioner/client relationship.

The pressures of modern living demand that we take more care of ourselves in an effort to remain healthy. However, despite our increased self-awareness and best endeavours to achieve optimum health, many of us still become ill. This is giving rise to deeper questioning and a willingness to understand why we are prone to disease in the first place.

HOW ILLNESS IS VIEWED
Changes are taking place in society's concept of illness. Smoking and excessive drinking are now firmly recognised as having a detrimental effect on our health. We are being

recommended to follow a sensible diet and to take more exercise. We are also becoming more aware of the effects that hereditary and environmental factors and pollution may have on many health problems. Increasingly, it is being acknowledged that many illnesses are stress-related. However, it is still the widely-held view that disease is caused or influenced by external factors, that it is recognised by specific names, and that symptoms are looked upon as unrelated events. Holistic practitioners, by contrast, view symptoms as a warning sign from our vital healing force that something is wrong on a deeper level. This subtle and scientifically undetectable healing force seeks constantly to protect and keep us in a state of balance. Disharmony, manifesting as illness, has an inner, psychological, emotional or spiritual cause and, until the dis-connection is addressed, complete healing cannot take place. To accept this premise requires a shift in understanding and an opportunity to embrace other possibilities.

BODY-MIND

To understand what the body-mind is, we have to turn around old patterns of thought and embrace the concept that there is a total unity and interdependence of our body, mind, spirituality and emotions. These human components are unique to each of us and constantly interact in an effort to bring balance and harmony to the whole.

We have been given the responsibility of our own health and the facility of an inner doctor to enable us to heal ourselves. In the way that we understand the dialogue of the body-mind and approach our illness, we hold the key to our own well-being.

TREATMENTS OFFERED

Knowing that we have the in-built facility of self-healing does not, of course, make conventional medicine redundant. However, we can make choices in our approach to assisted healing and it is useful to explore the fundamental differences offered by the scientific and natural systems.

For centuries, orthodox medicine has sought to cure by suppressing or removing the symptom diagnosed as the health problem, rather than looking at its cause. Following treatment, the underlying cause may, in the course of time, again make itself known by producing another more serious symptom. Renamed and re-treated, the inward progression of disease continues, creating greater pressure on the individual's system. Drugs are often administered indiscriminately, not seeming to acknowledge the patient's unique sensitivity.

The psychosomatic causes of disease, although raising more interest in recent years within the medical profession, are still largely ignored. On the whole, less emphasis is placed on the underlying attitude of patients and their reaction to stress. These are important factors in strengthening or weakening the immune system in its vital role of protecting the body. A positive attitude during times of illness can have a direct bearing on the effectiveness of any form of treatment; this is true in all therapies.

Conventional medicine, often prepared from the very same plants used in herbal therapies, extracts only the essence identified as being helpful to a particular illness. Natural therapists use the balanced value of the plant, or any part of it. In addition, they place greater emphasis on the therapeutic value of everyday foods.

There are many holistic remedies and therapies from

which to choose. Often similar in their approach or complementing each other, some can be combined whilst others are best used alone. When using self-help methods, it is not advisable to try everything at once. Natural methods often appear to work more slowly, so it is wise to have patience and try one thing at a time unless remedies are known to be compatible.

All natural therapists aim to stimulate the body to balance and heal itself. If you have difficulty in deciding which natural remedy or therapy to use, your way forward can often become clearer if you select that to which you feel drawn or in which you have a natural interest. You should also take care when choosing a practitioner that you sense a personal rapport and are satisfied with their qualifications and/or experience. Of prime importance to any therapist is the deeper meaning of the presenting problem. As the patient, you will be encouraged to participate in your healing and re-connection with your true self.

RELATING TO THE MENOPAUSE

The menopause presents an opportunity for women to establish this re-connection. It often comes at a time when women's energy levels and morale can be at a low ebb. Childbirth, rearing and caring for a family, coping with teenagers or adjusting to children leaving home for independent lives, juggling outside employment with home duties or managing successful careers, years of feeling drained by menstruation—all take their toll. The circumstances leading up to and following premature menopause in the case of hysterectomy often require a greater fortitude and degree of support.

Although each woman's experience of the menopause is

her own and different, the way in which she experiences it depends on the health of her body, mind and spirit. The aim for any woman should be:

(a) to understand the process

(b) to treat it as a shared experience and not feel alone

(c) to try to accept and take steps to ease the symptoms

(d) to pass through and emerge at the other end in a positive frame of mind, with a healthy active body and enhanced emotional awareness.

As a woman, you can choose to use your menopausal phase as a time of reflection, an opportunity to re-assess, develop and reap rewards. You can accept the challenge of using a greater understanding of your personal power and the wisdom within you to your own benefit and the benefit of those around you. The choice is yours.

CHAPTER THREE

HRT

WHAT IS **HRT?**

HRT or hormone replacement therapy can only be medically prescribed. It is made synthetically and is a substitute for oestrogen and progesterone, which are hormones produced in the body. Unacceptable side-effects experienced by some women as a result of oestrogen being given alone brought about the addition of progestogen, a synthetic form of progesterone. The treatment is now most often given as a combination of oestrogen and progestogen and is available in the form of pills, creams, patches and implants.

HRT was introduced to Britain from America in the late Seventies and has only been prescribed extensively here for fifteen years. Still in its infancy and the subject of much discussion and controversy, research into its action, side-effects and long-term safety continues.

CAN IT HELP?

Conventional medicine considers that menopausal symptoms are caused by a fall in oestrogen levels and, if appropriate for the patient, offers HRT to relieve symptoms. There is no doubt that HRT can often speedily arrest the symptoms of hot flushes/night sweats, stress incontinence and dryness of the vagina.

Evidence suggests that HRT can also help with osteoporosis (loss of bone density) if taken early enough. However, the treatment cannot replace lost bone. It is also useful to younger women who have had a total hysterectomy before the menopause begins, as this would put them in a high-risk category for osteoporosis. In addition, there is evidence that HRT can afford some protection to post-menopausal women against heart disease, because it may reduce cholesterol levels.

THE DOWNSIDE: IS IT SAFE?

Present evidence indicates that long-term use of HRT could possibly increase the incidence of cancer of the breast and womb. Certain women are not medically eligible to take HRT; it is not prescribed where there is a history of:

- fibroids and endometriosis (the presence of functioning endometrial tissue in an abnormal location, usually the ovary)
- diabetes, liver or gall-bladder disease and gallstones.

Or where there is a family history of:

- blood clots in the veins or lungs
- cancer of the breast.

Three separate research studies have recently confirmed that HRT carries a significant increased risk of blood clots forming in the lungs and legs. The increased risk (between two-fold and four-fold in cases of blood clots in the legs) is now considered to be higher than the risk associated with the use of oral contraceptives by younger women. It has been found that the risks are higher nearer commencement of treatment (as they are with the contraceptive pill) and in the first year of treatment. This throws into doubt the wisdom of using HRT in the short term. Experts can still give no indication of what the combined effect will be of taking HRT following the use of the contraceptive pill.

There is increasing concern, following a recent study commissioned by the Government, that sex hormones in sewage can cause sexual changes in carp and trout. This opens up the disturbing possibility that sex hormones could also be entering the water cycle, with no way to extract them known at present.

KNOWN SIDE-EFFECTS AND DRAWBACKS

Many women are deterred from taking HRT because of the risk of developing cancer or, as a result of experiencing side-effects, stop taking it within six months. Reported side-effects include:

- inconvenience of cyclical bleeding
- raised blood pressure
- depression
- symptoms often associated with pre-menstrual syndrome: irritability and mood swings, headaches, breast soreness, weight gain, fluid retention, nausea
- thrush
- varicose veins
- pains in the legs and cramps
- encouragement of the growth of fibroids
- vague symptoms of feeling unwell.

HRT depletes the body of vital vitamins and minerals and there is no evidence that it can help with the emotional symptoms of the menopause. It has been established that, for maximum protection against osteoporosis, HRT has to be taken for at least ten years.

Doubtless many women would be horrified to learn of the cruelty inflicted on pregnant mares in order to obtain their urine, which is used in the manufacture of some HRT drugs and of the fate of their unwanted foals who are removed from their mothers and fattened for slaughter. Those who are concerned about animal welfare should seek the cooperation of their doctors in being prescribed HRT not made from mares' urine.

WHAT IS THE APPEAL OF HRT?

The keenness of doctors to prescribe HRT and praise for it by some women in the public eye who take it, may persuade you that HRT is a wonder therapy. You may be convinced that, by taking it, you will immediately look and feel younger, enjoy an abundance of energy, possibly well into advanced old age, and even have a better sex life. You may view it as an elixir of youth and a panacea for good health. Reputable doctors will tell you that it should not be considered to be any such thing.

A HOLISTIC VIEW

Leaving aside the social pressures and possible lack of awareness of the holistic approach, the appeal of HRT raises some interesting points:

(a) Why are some women desperate to look younger?

(b) Why are they anxious to sweep their symptoms under the carpet and take the quick way out?

(c) Why do they get so upset because the body is slowing down, choosing to take treatment which they hope will make it function faster?

(d) What is the attraction of living now and maybe paying later?

In looking more deeply at the possible reasons for such

attitudes, you should consider whether there may be underlying emotional problems such as fear, lack of confidence or invalidation involved. Are you, perhaps, locked into the habit of caring for others or of carrying on regardless? Are you ignoring the need to make time for your own personal nourishment?

If you constantly overwork, prefer to stay in the fast lane and go to any lengths to retain a youthful appearance, you should, perhaps, stop to ask yourself why you feel the need to carry on proving yourself and to whom? Taking HRT allows women to remain stuck in their old patterns of behaviour. On an energy level, it is impossible to tackle buried issues and move forward through the menopause to what could be a brighter time ahead.

Drug companies have a huge financial investment in HRT. They need to push it hard, using clever marketing techniques and exerting pressure on doctors to prescribe their products. In passing over the management of their health to drug companies, women are being exploited and used as guinea pigs. Their fears and shortcomings are being played upon for financial gain. Most of the current research into the menopause is funded and carried out by the drug companies. There continues to be a big question mark over the safety of HRT: it is being prescribed before the long-term effects are known. Remember, these drugs are invasive, powerful, synthetically made substances, which have a profound effect on the entire system. They can often produce symptoms never experienced before. *Ironically, even more profit can be made from the sale of drugs to counteract the side-effects of HRT.*

The body is self-regulating and becomes confused and thrown out of balance when extra oestrogen is taken. In being forced to work at a pace which is undesirable, the body then slows down or permanently stops its production of natural oestrogen. In endeavouring to deal with a complex problem, medicine is adopting the over-simplified approach of singling out the sex hormones for treatment. This can have a far-reaching effect on the body's vital force and fine balance. HRT does not touch the core of a woman and the more subtle aspects of her make-up. It suppresses symptoms, making it impossible to address the causes. Symptoms are a 'gift'. They provide an opportunity for women to get in touch with themselves—to explore and deal with the messages they give and re-build good health.

There are plenty of gentle, low-cost, holistic measures which can be taken to build and maintain good health and encourage the balanced production of essential natural hormones. Many menopausal problems, including osteo-porosis, are preventable or could be treated by making changes to diet and lifestyle. It is important to build strong bones before the mid-thirties. One of the best ways of doing this is to use your limbs and take regular exercise. Weak bones were not a problem for primitive humans and are not a problem to women today in many cultures where they naturally use their legs to walk and work and have a healthy diet and lifestyle. Factors such as stress, the prolonged use of steroids, smoking, too much alcohol, a diet high in protein, fat and processed food and low in calcium should be recognised as contributing to bone loss.

There are recognised herbs to build strong bones. Recently, Natural Progesterone (an organic preparation derived from the wild yam) has been found to have the same effect. Therapies such as homoeopathy and Chinese medicine are also of enormous value.

It is important to remember that HRT is not a contraceptive treatment. If you start taking it before your periods have naturally ended, you could still become pregnant. It is normally recommended that contraceptive measures are used for a year after the last period. If you are uncertain about the need to continue contraception at the time of menopause, seek medical advice.

If you are considering taking HRT, or if your symptoms are so severe that you think there is no alternative, look at as much information as possible to help you make an informed choice. Take advantage of the expertise of practitioners before deciding whether the treatment is for you. If you are already taking HRT and wish to stop, it is important to remember that this should be done under medical supervision. Sudden discontinuation of the treatment can make symptoms worse.

To sum up, the holistic view is that there is no need to re-arrange the course of nature. If you are willing to move with the flow of life, accepting and adapting to the changes it brings, you can gracefully enter and enjoy a tranquil new phase. You can take responsibility for yourself and, in so doing, recognise that your body—given the care appropriate to its needs—is designed to maintain good health and balance. You can then work towards a better and healthier future for yourself and the generations to come.

CHAPTER FOUR

Natural Progesterone

THE ROLES OF OESTROGEN AND PROGESTERONE IN THE BODY

The beginning of puberty brings the hormone oestrogen into play in a woman's body. Sexual organs mature, female characteristics develop and menstruation begins. The ovaries start working, making oestrogen for the first ten or eleven days of the menstrual cycle; this stimulates the building up of a bloody lining in the womb in anticipation of a pregnancy. Every woman is born with around 300,000 partially developed eggs (follicles). At the point in the menstrual cycle when a follicle releases the egg, the body switches over to making the progesterone hormone. (This only happens when ovulation is occurring.) Progesterone ensures that the lining of the womb is held in place and also has the function of stopping the other ovary from producing an egg. It has a balancing effect on oestrogen and protects a woman's body from its side-effects.

In the natural course of events, oestrogen falls into a decline at menopause. It is, however, still produced to a lesser extent in other glands of the body, the adrenals having an important function in this continuing process. Although production of progesterone ceases when ovulation no longer occurs, nature has provided plants and foods which have a progestogenic effect, helping women stay in balance for longer.

SYNTHETIC PROGESTERONE

During the 1960s, the pharmaceutical companies, already aware of the benefits of progesterone treatment, turned their attention from researching the sources of the progesterone-like molecule in the plant kingdom to patenting, manufacturing and marketing a saleable, synthetic product. Synthetic progesterone—progestogen or progestin—has risen in popularity with the medical profession and the public in recent times. This is because of its ease of use as a contraceptive and value in protecting against the oestrogen-induced risk of cancer of the womb and many other serious conditions.

A product not found in the natural world can be patented and owned, with sales and prices being controlled by the owner. It is a route to profit. Pharmaceutical companies are reluctant to spend large sums of money researching a natural product when a competitor could produce the same product with little outlay.

Some companies making progestogens have large farms in Mexico, where they cultivate the 'wild' yam, extracting from it the sterol diosgenin, which is easily converted into natural progesterone. This substance is then converted into something very similar, which can conveniently be taken by mouth, unlike the natural product previously used which was administered by injection. In the process of making the synthetic product, the molecular structure is changed; it does not act in the same way in the body as its natural counterpart and produces a wide range of side-effects.

There is an alarmingly long list of warnings and contra-indications relating to major health problems attributed to progestogens. These include cancer of the breast and womb, liver dysfunction and blood clotting. In addition, there are many reported undesirable side-effects, such as: imbalance in calcium, glucose and insulin levels, appearance of unwanted facial hair, fluid retention; depletion of vitamins and minerals, weight gain, skin problems, depression, headaches, dizziness, insomnia, breast tenderness, fatigue, breakthrough bleeding and cystitis.

Progestogens carry a warning that their use by pregnant women can kill the baby or cause congenital malformation. Their function is the opposite of natural progesterone, which is necessary for the baby's survival in the womb.

NATURAL PROGESTERONE AND DR JOHN LEE

The alarming increase during the mid-seventies in the number of women developing osteoporosis, its earlier onset and problems associated with its treatment using synthetic hormones, left the medical profession lacking a positive solution.

In 1979, John Lee, a family doctor practising in California, heard a talk given by biochemist Professor Ray Peat, who was seeking to re-educate his medical colleagues on the benefits of natural progesterone, obtainable from the wild yam root, and its key physiological role in the body. Professor Peat put forward the advantages of using a natural progesterone cream which could be easily absorbed by the skin.

The talk struck a responsive chord in Dr Lee. He decided to offer Cielo (now Pro-Gest), a progesterone cream sold over the counter in the United States and originally marketed as a skin moisturiser, to patients with menopausal osteoporosis who were precluded from taking oestrogen because of contra-indications such as a history of cancer of the breast or womb. The availability locally of a new technique for measuring bone density enabled accurate information to be obtained on the condition of these patients' bones. Amazing increases in bone density were confirmed within six to twelve months of patients using the cream. *This had never been recorded in medical history before.*

These women were also reporting many other improvements in their health: increased energy and general well-being, recovery from mild hypothyroidism, a lowering of blood pressure in those previously having mild symptoms and a return of libido. There was also a bonus—no side-effects.

Dr Lee decided to extend his user base of natural progesterone cream to women who were already taking oestrogen. Soon after commencing treatment, some of this group of women developed various symptoms: breast tenderness, fluid retention and spotting. This was the result of the progesterone making them more sensitive to the oestrogen in their bodies. The lesson Dr Lee learned from this was that the oestrogen dose should be cut in half when starting natural progesterone treatment, and gradually reduced, with the aim of eventual discontinuation.

More almost unbelievably good results emerged from this group of patients. Problems with the unwanted growth of facial hair and thinning of scalp hair reversed; diuretics became unnecessary, as did blood pressure pills because, without the water retention, the blood pressure normalised. Similarly, the natural progesterone helped reactivate sluggish thyroid function and thyroid medication also became unnecessary.

Many herbs and everyday foods contain progesterone or possess progesterone precursors. Amongst the best-known of these is mistletoe. Several years before attending Professor Peat's lecture, Dr Lee had already taken an interest in natural progesterone while investigating the European mistletoe for a medical magazine article. During his research, he discovered that a myriad of health benefits were attributed to the plant in many different cultures in the world. Kissing under the mistletoe is a reminder of a much older tradition. During pre-Christian festivities at the winter solstice, heated wine was laced with mistletoe berries. We are now aware that, among other things, progesterone increases libido, brings feelings of well-being and has contraceptive properties, so it is not difficult to imagine how useful it was at a time of merriment and possibly free sexual licence. At the end of the festival week, ceasing to drink the wine laced with mistletoe berries would have encouraged the onset of a period in menstruating women, dealing with the problem of any unwanted pregnancies.

Native women of the Trobriand islands (off Papua New Guinea) do not experience the menopausal symptoms which Western society has come to accept as the norm. The birth rate is low and islanders are happy, healthy, lead active sex lives and are not overweight. Their diet is fresh and natural, the staple food being the wild yam (not the same as the sweet potato), which Dr Lee believes contains progesterone precursors or progesterone itself.

Absence of menopausal symptoms is found in many other cultures in the world — all having the common factors of lack of oestrogen dominance coupled with a natural, healthy diet and lifestyle. Recognising that there are many factors involved in creating a smooth passage through menopause and maintaining good health thereafter, Dr Lee is keen that women support their use of natural progesterone cream with dietary and lifestyle adjustments. (In raising the general level of health, the beneficial effects of the natural hormone will be enhanced.) Full details of his osteoporosis treatment programme are given in his book, *Natural Progesterone— The Multiple Roles of a Remarkable Hormone.*

Dr Lee has now retired from medical practice. He continues to lecture at home and abroad and is writing further books on natural progesterone. It is to his everlasting credit that his pioneering spirit and tireless efforts eventually overcame red tape and resistance, enabling important research findings to be brought to the attention of the medical establishment and general public. He can also take satisfaction from the fact that he has made great inroads in re-educating the medical profession on the central role progesterone plays in the chemistry of the body and its overwhelming benefits when applied in a natural form. Public demand for his cream and its results speak for themselves.

Dr Lee has also played a significant part in alerting the public to the almost epidemic problem of oestrogen bombardment in our society today. Significant changes are needed to overcome this.

USING NATURAL PROGESTERONE CREAM

Natural progesterone cream should be applied to areas of the body where the skin is thin. The progesterone molecule is fat soluble; thicker skin would hinder effective absorption. Suitable skin sites are the face (test a small area first), behind the ears, the neck, upper chest, abdomen and inside of the arms and thighs. Twice daily application of the cream should be rotated—one day use one arm, the next day the other. Do not return to the same skin site within four to five days. Beneficial reaction will vary from person to person, so it may be one to three months before full improvements are felt.

USING NATURAL PROGESTERONE CREAM WITH SYNTHETIC HORMONES

If you wish to use natural progesterone cream and are already taking HRT (combined oestrogen and progestogen) with a view to discontinuing, Dr Lee recommends that you taper the dose of synthetics over a three-month period, cutting the dose by half each month. You may, however, wish to remain on a very low dose of HRT.

AVAILABILITY OF NATURAL PROGESTERONE CREAM

Natural progesterone cream is at present classed as an unlicensed medicine in the United Kingdom and cannot be purchased without a prescription. However, there are a growing number of doctors who are prescribing natural progesterone cream; a few will prescribe on the NHS, but the majority have to be consulted privately.

WILD YAM EXTRACT

Creams containing the extract of wild yam are now available over the counter in the UK. However, their action is different from natural progesterone cream and will not have the same effect. Wild yam extract should only be taken by mouth, for example in tincture form.

FURTHER INFORMATION ON NATURAL PROGESTERONE CREAM

The Natural Progesterone Information Service in Sussex provides information packs, books, audio tapes, a video and a list of doctors in the UK prescribing natural progesterone cream. It does not advise any woman to use a hormone, even a non-toxic one, without consulting a doctor who can monitor her progress. The natural progesterone cream recommended by The Natural Progesterone Information Service and Dr John Lee is Pro-Gest. (Dr Lee has no financial interest in this company.) See Useful Addresses for contact details.

CHAPTER FIVE

Aromatherapy

WHAT IS AROMATHERAPY?

Aromatherapy uses the powerful healing properties of fragrant plant oils—mostly obtained by steam distillation to create intensely concentrated essential oils—derived from a vast variety of aromatic herbs, roots, grasses, woods, fruits, berries, spices, leaves and flowers which grow in every corner of our earth. Many thousands of years old, aromatherapy is a vital element in the numerous plant-based healing traditions which reveal the natural world as a place of abundant miracles, if we just have the eyes to see and the hearts, minds and humility to respect and understand. Through its essential oils we receive the healing energies of the sun, earth, air and rain—gathered and transformed by the living plant.

SOME BACKGROUND

Aromatic essences have been used throughout human history; indeed, the word 'perfume' derives from the Latin *per fumare* meaning 'to smoke through'; this reveals the ancient custom of burning aromatic branches and leaves to drive away the evil spirits that were thought to cause infection and psychological malaise. In the early years of this century, juniper, thyme and rosemary were still smoked on fires in French cottage hospitals to limit airborne infection.

The Ancient Egyptians used aromatics steeped in animal fats as medicines, as cosmetics and to vapourise during religious ritual to induce altered states of consciousness. At the time of Christ's birth they were so highly valued that Frankincense and Myrrh were offered along with gold to the infant Jesus. Today, whilst many aromatic plants yield relatively copious amounts of oil and are widely grown, others—especially the wonderful flower oils such as Rose, Jasmine and Orange blossom (Neroli)—command a price similar to that of pure gold, reflecting the vast acreage of plant material needed to produce tiny quantities of essential oil.

WHAT ARE ESSENTIAL OILS?

In aromatic plants, essential oils play a similar role to the hormones produced by our own endocrine glands: maintaining and normalising thousands of physiological processes. Extraordinarily complex and subtle in their structure, they possess a huge range of therapeutic effects, making them helpful to just about any need—whether physical or emotional. Being compatible with our own skin oils and intracellular fluids, and having molecules which enable them to pass through the epidermis and very fine lung surfaces, they rapidly enter the entire bloodstream. Inhaled, they directly access the limbic area of the brain, which governs all our essential emotional responses and memories.

We can, perhaps, begin to see how aromatherapy is uniquely placed to help and to heal us at the level where our bodies, minds and feelings interweave and from which our true health and well-being arises.

AROMATHERAPY IN PRACTICE

Aromatherapy can vary in application according to the preference and experience of the practitioner. Many aromatherapists are trained in other skills such as nursing, nutrition, counselling, reflexology, Swedish massage and shiatsu. Generally, you should expect that a treatment will last between one and one and a half hours, with an additional period initially to ask about your health, medical background, lifestyle, main stresses and how you would like aromatherapy to help you. This facilitates the choice of a small number of the most appropriate essential oils which are blended in a carrier oil and applied to the body, limbs, hands, feet, head and face. Aromatherapy massage is wonderfully gentle, yet amazingly powerful. At the end of your treatment, you will be left to rest for a while in warmth and comfort.

Most aromatherapists will encourage you to use essential oils at home as an important way of enhancing your treatments—the self-help use of the oils forms a major part of aromatherapy. Because the essential oils are very powerful, it is vital to have and to follow sound advice and information on their use. It is also important to buy good quality, unadulterated essential oils such as Tisserand, which is available in many good health food stores or by mail order, and Swanfleet, which is available by mail order only. Celia Hewson, the aromatherapist advisor for this book, highly recommends the products supplied mail order by the partnership of Norman and Germaine Rich. Quantities are usually 25ml and upwards, but the more expensive oils can be purchased in smaller quantities. (See Useful Addresses.)

FINDING A PRACTITIONER

The quality and length of aromatherapy training varies enormously and is not currently regulated by legislation. You are strongly advised to contact the International Federation of Aromatherapists (see Useful Addresses). It sets the standard in training and research and produces a nationwide list of its full members on request.

AROMATHERAPY AND THE MENOPAUSE

It is important to understand that the menopause is intended by nature to be a gentle transition from your reproductive years to a new and fulfilling phase of life. Aromatherapy is a powerful ally in ensuring that you experience these years and the future in just this way. As you receive the healing energies of essential oils, you can come to know that you are truly the co-creator of your own well-being.

The huge range of essential oils means that hundreds of different blends or single oils can be applied to problems arising during the menopause. In general though, the following guidelines apply.

HORMONAL BALANCERS

Rose The essential oil most closely associated with the female reproductive system and the hormonal activity which regulates it. Rose has a powerful cleansing and balancing effect on the uterus and is excellent for irregular or excessive menstrual flow. It enhances confidence in the feminine self and can help to restore diminished libido.

Geranium By stimulating the adrenal cortex, Geranium regulates female reproductive hormones. Its effect is tonic and normalising for the whole system and its diuretic and circulation stimulating action reduces fluid retention.

Lavender The essential oil with the widest range of therapeutic qualities; it regulates the endocrine and nervous systems. Its action is calming and balancing for the whole range of menstrual and menopausal symptoms.

Basil Another stimulator of hormones produced by the adrenal cortex which regulate female sex hormones. Balances scanty and painful periods.

Sage Contains powerful plant oestrogens which regulate excessive menstrual flow. Should be avoided by epilepsy sufferers. Should only be used in tiny amounts and best used under advice from a qualified aromatherapist (see Toxicity, p. 37).

Thyme A powerful stimulant, physically and mentally. Improves painful and irregular periods, fluid retention, poor circulation and fatigue. The gentler form of Thyme Linolol, avoids problems with skin irritation.

Cypress A high plant oestrogen content gives it excellent affinity with the female reproductive and endocrine system. It is astringent, balancing and antispasmodic (relieves muscle spasms, tension and abdominal cramps), easing painful and excessive menstruation, menopausal spotting and fluid retention.

Note Plant oestrogens are generally weaker than their powerful synthetic chemical counterparts and, by binding to the body's oestrogen receptors, actually help to balance oestrogen levels.

NERVOUS SYSTEM REGULATORS
Calming

Vetivert With its deep, woody aroma, reminiscent of tree roots in damp earth, it has a uniquely grounding effect on the nervous system—helping to dissolve extreme tension and anxiety and to facilitate sound sleep.

Petitgrain Its slightly smoky citrus aroma is strengthening and tonic to the nervous system. Petitgrain eases palpitations, anxiety and insomnia.

Lavender Balancing, strengthening and calming to the nervous system. It reduces high blood pressure.

Ylang Ylang Calms and regulates the nervous system. It helps in cases of anxiety, shock, anger, palpitations, rapid heartbeat and high blood pressure. Its euphoric effect on the emotions makes it an excellent anti-depressant.

Sweet Marjoram Its powerful aroma is warming and strengthening emotionally. A deeply calming essential oil, it eases anxiety, depression and insomnia. (Also excellent for muscle and joint aches and pains.)

Clary Sage Euphoric and calming at the same time. An excellent muscle relaxant. Avoid using before driving and when drinking alcohol.

Neroli Its beautiful orange blossom aroma provides a gentle sedative, which is anti-depressant and restores emotional and sexual confidence. It strengthens and calms the nervous system and eases palpitations and insomnia.

Roman Chamomile A supremely soothing, anti-inflammatory oil, both physically and emotionally, it helps overcome anxiety, irritability and nervousness.

Uplifting

Bergamot With its warm and fresh citrusy aroma, it gives a real lift to the spirits. It is grounding, anti-tension and anti-depressant. Helps to restore lost appetite.

Geranium Supremely balancing, it moderates extremes of emotion and is uplifting, tonic and anti-depressant.

Frankincense Enhances your ability to breathe deeply and is very strengthening if you are fearful, experiencing sleep broken by nightmares, or releasing old emotions.

Jasmine Its powerful and beautiful aroma is warming and stimulating. It releases blocked, 'hardened' emotions with its euphoric and aphrodisiac qualities. Resolves fatigue associated with depression.

Juniper Extremely strengthening and cleansing, it protects against your own and others' negative emotions. Good for mental and physical sluggishness.

Lavender Both tonic and calming, lavender balances the mind and emotions against extremes—as in fluctuating moods, manic depression and hysteria.

Orange A very uncomplicated, cheering oil, with its bright citrus scent. Helps to resolve insomnia.

Rosemary A powerful mental and nervous system tonic, it clears the mind, strengthens the memory and offers courage, clarity and purposefulness. An excellent reliever of pain, especially when blended with Lavender.

Tangerine An excellent, gentle nerve tonic with its high vitamin C content. It is uplifting whilst also settling. Well known as a children's remedy, it also helps you to get in touch with your own inner child—your deep emotional needs.

Ylang Ylang Yet another example of how essential oils can have apparently paradoxical effects; it calms the mind and yet has a euphoric and confidence-boosting action. Its aroma is very sweet and floral and so is best balanced with a citrus oil, such as Bergamot.

Rose Helps you to contact and maintain your true feminine essence. It restores confidence and libido and lifts depression, whilst maintaining calm feelings.

Basil An excellent nerve tonic, which provides courage and clear-headedness. A remedy for mental fatigue and nervous debility.

Lemon Refreshing, relaxing and strengthening for the nervous system.

Peppermint Regulates the nervous system. It clears the head and confused thoughts. Gives a feeling of freshness, clarity and brightness. Is excellent to inhale for shock.

Clary Sage Euphoric and creates a heightened state of mind to counter depression, while being powerfully relaxant.

Thyme An excellent nervous system tonic. Small amounts will relieve insomnia while it also lifts fatigue and enlivens those needing to feel more wakeful.

Digestives

Basil Good antispasmodic, which eases heartburn, especially when associated with mental fatigue and tension.

Bergamot Restores appetite by resolving anxiety and possibly by affecting appetite control mechanisms.

Roman Chamomile Gently anti-spasmodic and anti-inflammatory, it relieves the sharp pains of irritable bowel syndrome, heartburn, excess acidity and ulcers.

Sweet Marjoram Warming, anti-spasmodic and pain relieving, it eases griping pain and constipation and strengthens proper intestinal function.

Ginger Warming and tonic, it eases constipation, but also eases diarrhoea when of a cold, mucusy type.

Black Pepper Very warming and stimulant for a sluggish digestive system, but without sending it into spasm.

Orange Regulates and tones the entire digestive tract to overcome nausea and constipation.

Lemon Very tonic and cleansing—especially for the liver and gall-bladder. It helps to metabolise fats and resolve anaemia.

Peppermint An excellent liver tonic, it relieves nausea and indigestion. Has an excellent antiseptic and antispasmodic effect for the intestinal wall muscles: peppermint oil capsules are often prescribed for irritable bowel and diverticulosis.

Sage Very purifying and anti-bacterial, with an antispasmodic effect when used in small amounts; but beware its toxic potential and its ability to provide severe spasm if overused.

Thyme Strengthens the intestinal wall muscles. Thyme has an anti-bacterial effect and stimulates sluggish digestion.

You will find a selection of 'recipes' formulated by an experienced aromatherapist to treat specific menopause conditions in Chapter 16 Common Symptoms and Holistic Treatments. However, if you wish to choose oils for yourself, generally you will achieve much better results by working on just one set of symptoms at a time until improvement is found—especially when combining a bath and body oil treatment. It is, on the other hand, fine to work on, say, varicose veins while also treating a burning mouth or dizziness, as there is no overlap or duplication of methods. Avoid using more than four oils together, as doing this might produce a 'muddy'-smelling blend and be less effective therapeutically.

With the exception of the very expensive oils of Rose, Jasmine and Neroli, essential oils retail at between £3-£15 for 5-15ml quantities. Expect to pay more for true Chamomile.

USING ESSENTIAL OILS

The following provides enough information for you to begin using essential oils safely at home.

All essential oils should be kept in tightly closed dark glass bottles in a cool, shaded place and will last for at least two years. Citrus oils are at their best for six months only and essential oils mixed in a carrier oil for two months. Essential oils for bath and body can be dispensed or blended direct from their individual bottles each time you wish to use them.

For greater convenience, especially if you are using an identical blend to treat an ongoing condition which may be required daily over one to three months, mix the oils for both bath and body use as a concentrate in a 10ml dropper bottle—obtainable from any chemist. The concentrate method has several advantages, including:

- ease of use where this is daily or prolonged, as the drops can be immediately dispensed
- it avoids taking several bottles into the warm atmosphere of the bathroom and constantly exposing the oils to oxidation, which could cause deterioration
- greater safety, as the pipette mechanism of the dropper bottle is more controllable than most plastic inserts (fitted in many essential oil bottles), which can become blocked or allow a sudden out-rush of oils
- keeps the user focused on dealing with one problem at a

time, rather than flitting from blend to blend
- achieves better synergy between the essential oils and more subtle blends. (Synergy is a blend of two or more essential oils, which alters their joint properties when combined and has a more powerful and dynamic effect than using them together singly.)

When using larger quantities of drops in the preparation of a stock concentrate, ensure as far as possible that you will not be disturbed. It might help to make a written note when you have added the required number of drops from each bottle of essential oil. Whichever method you use, always remember to replace the caps on bottles containing essential oil straight away. The quantities of drops for both the above methods are given, where applicable, in Chapter 16.

AROMATIC BATHS

Run a warm bath and turn off the taps. Immediately before getting in, mix a total of six to eight drops of essential oil into the water. (Mixing them first in a little full fat milk improves dispersal.) Soak for ten to fifteen minutes, relaxing and inhaling deeply before using any soaps, etc. When first treating an ongoing problem, take a daily aromatic bath (day or evening for relaxing blends; up to about 7 pm for more stimulating oils). Reduce to three or four baths weekly as your condition improves.

BODY OILS

A good general concentration for healthy adults is two and a half per cent—occasionally stronger for very small, localised areas. To achieve this, buy a 50ml bottle of sweet almond oil from a pharmacy and add thirty drops of your chosen essential oils to it, shaking well. Apply sparingly, especially when the skin is damp after your bath or shower.

FACE OILS, CREAMS, LOTIONS

It is best to use an unperfumed cream, lotion base or jojoba which nourishes the skin without over-feeding it. Mix ten drops of your chosen essential oils thoroughly into 50g or 50ml of base to produce a concentration of one per cent.

COMPRESSES

In the context of this book, these will usually be hot compresses to relieve pain and spasm, as in dyspepsia or abdominal cramps. Pour very hot water into a bowl or basin and drop six to eight drops of essential oils onto the surface. Using a small, nappy-sized towel or cloth, dip into the surface, wring out any excess water and immediately place on the area to be treated. Leave in place until it completely loses its heat, reapplying every half hour if necessary until the pain eases.

INHALATIONS

Drop three to four drops of essential oils onto a tissue to inhale; or six to eight drops into a purchased diffuser or burner to perfume a room.

CAUTIONS

Whilst aromatherapy can offer much, the following people would be wise to avoid its use, except on the specific recommendations of a qualified and experienced aromatherapist:

- pregnant women, especially during the first three months

- babies, toddlers and children
- people with medical conditions such as epilepsy, cancer, heart or kidney and liver disease; also the frail and elderly.

REMEMBER:

- to keep your bottles of essential oils out of the reach of children, preferably in a locked cupboard
- not to use the essential oils or diluted blends in or near the eyes and to avoid rubbing the eyes until the hands are washed after touching the essential oils
- that although it can be an effective therapeutic method to take the oils by mouth under qualified supervision, you are advised to avoid this as severe damage can be caused to the digestive tract. There is, indeed, much evidence to show that just as much is effectively absorbed into the body by application of oils to the skin
- that under no circumstances should the amounts of essential oil stated be exceeded. This will *not* make them more therapeutically active.

  Some essential oils—e.g. Basil and Peppermint—are very strong and may cause skin irritation in other than tiny amounts or well diluted in a carrier oil. Cedarwood, Sage and Rosemary should be avoided by epileptics and Rosemary, Sage and Thyme by those with high blood pressure. Bergamot and other citrus oils can make the skin more photosensitive and so should be avoided before exposure to the sun.

TOXICITY

Some essential oils are hazardous because they may cause systemic poisoning or skin reactions. None of these is included in this book and a responsible aromatherapist will neither use nor recommend them. They include such oils as Pennyroyal, Wintergreen and Mugwort (Armoise). Common Sage can be relatively toxic if used in too great a quantity and/or too frequently and is best left to the qualified aromatherapist to apply; many prefer to use the similar therapeutic qualities of the safer Clary Sage.

Of the oils recommended here in blends, Lemon and Thyme can be somewhat toxic if used over a long period. White Thyme or, better still, the much gentler Thyme Linolol, are preferable to Red Thyme, which can be over-stimulating and damaging to the skin and liver.

No essential oil should be used continuously for longer than three weeks. If you need to treat specific symptoms beyond that time, take a break of at least one week and then either resume use for another three weeks or introduce an alternative blend for that condition. Anything which is used for longer than six weeks tends to become less effective as the body becomes accustomed to it.

Note It is advisable to seek medical advice if symptoms persist or worsen.

CASE HISTORIES

ROSALIE

At forty-eight, Rosalie had recently set up home with her partner—a kind, supportive man. Her daughter of fifteen lived with them and her partner's son of sixteen often visited at weekends and during the holidays. Having two failed marriages behind her, Rosalie was making a great effort to make everything perfect.

Rosalie had noticed that her menstrual cycle was

lengthening. This did not worry her as she was aware that it often happened at the time of menopause. However, she was upset by a deterioration in her emotional state. Her mood swings were very noticeable at home and at work. She felt like Jekyll and Hyde.

Rosalie's working life was stressful. She worked in a very busy shop and had a poor relationship with her boss. She found herself reacting even more to his unpleasant attitude. She often experienced panic attacks, causing her to feel shaky, weepy and breathless. Eventually, Rosalie's general practitioner insisted that she take at least two weeks off work, diagnosing 'nervous debility'.

Rosalie consulted an aromatherapist and decided to take advantage of this opportunity for a complete rest. As well as regular massage, Rosalie was given very sedative essential oils of Vetivert, Neroli, Chamomile, Rose Maroc and Sandalwood to use in the bath to help release her feelings of panic. She was also advised to massage a single undiluted drop of this blend anti-clockwise into her solar plexus, combined with deep breathing, before going to sleep and at any other time she started to feel shaky.

As Rosalie began to feel calmer and stronger, the aromatherapist changed to lighter oils which would maintain the more positive feelings, Lavender and Petitgrain for the bath and as a body oil. When she returned to work, Rosalie burned Geranium and Basil essential oils at home during the day or early evening. She also put some on a tissue at work to keep her mood positive and her mind clear and courageous so that she could tackle relationship issues which needed resolving.

Rosalie managed to obtain supportive part-time assistance in the shop and now feels less pressured. The panic attacks and mood swings have not recurred and Rosalie feels she is living happily ever after.

JOAN

Joan was fifty, happily married and working as a mobile hairdresser. Her main concerns were varicose veins and fluid retention in her legs and feet. As much of her work involved standing, she was experiencing a fair amount of discomfort.

Having been helped by aromatherapy in the past, Joan returned for consultation. The aromatherapist advised that strong lymphatic drainage massage was unsuitable due to the fragility of the veins, so much of her treatment focused on massage of the hip, buttocks and abdominal areas to remove congestion; this was partly caused by constipation, which was hampering circulation. Reflexology pressure points in her feet were also massaged to improve the function of the entire body. Essential oils of Rosemary, Lemon and Fennel (alternating with Black Pepper) were used as Joan is a chilly person, but had no problems with high blood pressure.

Joan was given an oil containing essential oils of Rosemary, Cypress, Lemon and Lavender to use at home twice daily, smoothing it into the abdomen, hips, buttocks, legs and feet, to improve the circulation and strength of the vein walls and to reduce scarring. She was advised to rest for at least fifteen minutes daily with her legs above head height—in this case by lying on her bed with pillows under her head and lower back for support, with her feet on the headboard. In addition, she was asked to increase the amount of fibre in her diet from fresh fruits and vegetables and low gluten wholegrains such as millet, brown rice and buckwheat and to drink plenty of mineral water rather than tea or coffee. Joan was also asked to reduce or avoid meat and dairy products. Vitamins C and E were taken daily to strengthen the veins.

After two months, Joan was happy to see and feel improvement. She can now carry out her work without discomfort. She has continued to eat a wholefood diet, feels much better and no longer suffers from constipation.

ALISON

Alison, aged forty-eight, was intelligent and strikingly beautiful. The director of a charity and of independent means, she lived with a much younger partner.

Alison was upset to find that she was experiencing unpleasant menopausal symptoms. Being a firm believer in alternative medicine, she had no wish to take HRT. When she consulted an aromatherapist, she was suffering from severe hot flushes and night sweats. She would often feel sick and dizzy if having to stand for any length of time, for example in a supermarket queue.

As she did little work outside the home, Alison was encouraged to increase the amount of rest and relaxation she allowed herself, including an hour's rest after lunch each day so that her nervous system would not always be on alert and upset her hormonal balance. She was also able to have weekly aromatherapy massage for six weeks using alternating blends of essential oils of Lavender, Rose, Geranium, Clary Sage and Cypress, aimed at calming and balancing the nervous and endocrine systems. A body oil was given, based on essential oils of Rose, Ylang Ylang and Bergamot, as the experience of menopause made her fear she would become less feminine and attractive to her partner. This she used after a daily bath with Lavender and Peppermint for their cooling effect.

Alison was delighted at the relief obtained and the speedy improvement in her symptoms.

CHAPTER SIX

The Bach Flower Remedies

AN INTRODUCTION

The fundamental principle behind Bach Flower remedies is that prolonged or acute emotional stress can give rise to debility and illness. The remedies are used to treat a particular type of person, a state of mind or mood. Their function is to address and gently cleanse negative emotions such as fear, worry, resentment and depression, enabling balance and harmony to be restored in the individual. The body is then in a position to concentrate on regaining optimum health and achieve its true potential.

THE CREATION OF THE REMEDIES

Edward Bach (pronounced batch) was born in Birmingham in 1896 of Welsh ancestry. From an early age, the exceptionally compassionate side of his nature was apparent and he knew that he wanted to be a doctor. He would dream of finding a simple form of healing which would cure all forms of illness. He would also dream that healing power would flow from his hands and that the sick would be healed; in fact he later developed and used this gift and was an effective 'hands on' healer.

Edward Bach had many sides to his nature—creatively and academically talented, he was independent, humorous, positive, selfless, kind and caring of all living things. He started his working life in his father's brass foundry, spent some time in the Yeomanry and started medical school at the age of twenty. Throughout his medical training, he had the sense that treating the physical symptoms was not enough and that other factors contributed to illness.

After qualifying as a doctor, Edward Bach moved into bacteriology and came into contact with homoeopathy. As a result of working on intestinal nosodes, he reached the same conclusions regarding the basic philosophy of homoeopathy as Samuel Hahnemann, its founder. He studied homoeopathy and practised this in addition to his medical work. Convinced that he should be treating the patient not the disease, he left his Harley Street practice in 1930. Armed with little more than a vision, a sense of purpose, his intuition and sensitivity, Dr Bach began his search for a simple, gentle, inexpensive form of healing, using the flowers of the countryside.

Wales was a place to which Edward Bach had returned many times when he had felt drawn to nature and his first remedy, Mimulus, was found there, though his search subsequently took him to many other places. Dr Bach discovered thirty-eight remedies, all but three made from wild flowers, which he said covered every negative state known to humankind. He was guided to identifying the particular flowers for each state by 'proving' their healing properties. He would experience moods, either after he had handled the flowers and the water in which they had been sitting in sunlight or prior to the remedy being found.

The following list of his remedies and brief descriptions are reproduced with the kind permission of The Dr Edward Bach Centre.

Agrimony Hides worries behind a brave face.

Aspen Apprehensive for no known reason.

Beech Critical and intolerant of others.

Century Weak-willed; exploited or imposed upon.

Cerato Doubts own judgment and seeks the confirmation of others.

Cherry Plum Uncontrolled, irrational thoughts, fear of mind giving way.

Chestnut Bud Refuses to learn by experience—continually repeats same mistakes.

Chicory Over-possessive, self-centred, clinging and over-protective, especially of loved ones.

Clematis Inattentive, dreamy, absent-minded, given to mental escapism.

Crab Apple (The 'Cleanser') Full of self disgust/detestation, ashamed of ailments.

Elm Overwhelmed by inadequacy and responsibility.

Gentian Despondent, easily discouraged, dejected from known cause.

Gorse Pessimistic, prone to defeatism, an 'Oh what's the use!' attitude.

Heather Talkative, obsessed with own troubles and experiences.

Holly Tendency towards hatred, envy, jealousy, suspicion.

Honeysuckle Tends to live in the past—nostalgic, home-sick.

Hornbeam Suffers from 'Monday morning' feeling—procrastination.

Impatiens Tendency towards impatience, irritability.

Larch Lacks self-confidence, feels inferior. Fears failure.

Mimulus Fears known things, shy, timid.

Mustard Feels saddened and low (under a 'dark cloud') for no known reason.

Oak Normally strong/courageous, but no longer able to struggle bravely against illness and/or adversity.

Olive Fatigued, drained of energy.

Pine Has guilt complex—blames self even for mistakes of others, always apologising.

Red Chestnut Obsessed by care and concern for others.

Rock Rose Suddenly alarmed, scared, panicky, suffers terror.

Rock Water Rigid minded, self-denying.

Scleranthus Shows uncertainty/indecision/vacillation, exhibits fluctuating moods.

Star of Bethlehem Exhibits after-effects of shock or trauma, great sorrow.

Sweet Chestnut Suffers utter dejection, a bleak outlook.

Vervain Over-enthusiastic—fanatical about beliefs, highly strung.

Vine Dominating/inflexible/tyrannical/autocratic/arrogant, usually a good leader.

Walnut Needing adjustment to transition or change, e.g. puberty, menopause, divorce, new surroundings.

Water Violet Proud, reserved, enjoys being alone.

White Chestnut Preoccupied with unwanted thoughts over problems or episodes, given to mental arguments.

Wild Oat Needing help in determining intended path in life.

Wild Rose Resigned, apathetic.

Willow Resentful, embittered, exhibits 'Poor old me' feelings.

Note More detailed descriptions of the remedies are contained in the books recommended in Helpful Reading.

After more than sixty years, the way the remedies are prepared remains the same. Twenty of the tinctures are prepared by the sunlight and water method. The rest are prepared by boiling. All are preserved in brandy.Dr Bach divided the thirty-eight states into seven groups, determined by his observations of human nature.These are:

• fear
• uncertainty
• lack of interest in the present
• loneliness
• over-caring for the welfare of others
• over-sensitive to influences and ideas
• despondency and despair.

After finding the thirty-eighth remedy, Dr Bach deemed the system complete. He had accomplished his vision, creating a method of healing which required no medical knowledge, enabling everyone—especially the poor and uneducated—to treat themselves. Five remedies were combined to form his now well-known Rescue Remedy for use in emergencies and acute problems: Cherry Plum, Clematis, Rock Rose, Impatiens and Star of Bethlehem.

Edward Bach's health deteriorated rapidly following the completion of his work. Sadly, he died in 1936 aged only fifty at Mount Vernon, Sotwell, Near Wallingford, his last home and the house from where he had set out to find many of the remedies. He left behind his system of healing, a small book, *The Twelve Healers and Other Remedies*, detailing his findings, and a small group of dedicated friends and companions who carried on his work. Mount Vernon is now the home of The Dr Edward Bach Centre, where the mother tinctures are still prepared and educational activities held. The staff seek to maintain the principles of this most rewarding therapy.

SELECTING REMEDIES FOR THE MENOPAUSE

When considering self-help measures for health problems occurring during the menopausal years, it is important to remember that the individual is viewed as a whole person and that treatment relates to the cause of the illness. When seeking to address the cause, you should take account of:

- your underlying type—indicated by your personality, outlook on life and reaction to stressful situations
- your prevailing mood/s and emotional state
- the guideline (also the golden rule in homoeopathy) to view the individual rather like an onion. This means that, in peeling back the outer layers, the obvious and easily observed problems should be treated first, leaving the deeper issues held in the inner layers to reveal themselves for attention when they are ready.

Greater benefits will be felt if the remedies chosen correspond as closely as possible to your personal picture. Endeavour to be honest with yourself when making a self-appraisal, even though you might prefer to disregard states which are undesirable or acceptable. It might be useful to ask someone who knows you well for their view of you. It is preferable to limit the selection of remedies to no more than six in one treatment.

CONSULTING A PRACTITIONER

A trained Bach practitioner will initially ensure that you, the client, are aware of what the therapy is intended to achieve and the confidential nature of the consultation. Adhering to the general principles of counselling, the practitioner will listen with empathy to your problems, observing pointers— apparent or offered in conversation—as a guide to your nature and feelings. Providing encouragement and reassurance, the practitioner's aim is to help you understand the deeper meaning of your problems, facilitating your participation in self-healing. He or she will discuss the selection of remedies with you in a positive way, offering another appointment when appropriate. Remedies are given in a 30ml treatment bottle.

TREATING YOURSELF
Widely available from health food stores and some chemists, the remedies/tinctures are sold in 10ml bottles. Remedies selected are normally prepared for treatment either by:
(a) adding two drops of each remedy to a glass of still mineral water to be sipped during the course of the day. This method is more suitable for emergency use or moods arising from temporary situations.
(b) filling a 30ml treatment/dropper bottle with still mineral water and adding two drops of the remedies chosen.

Four drops should be taken on the tongue four times daily, or more often if required. This method is economical and suitable for long-term use relating to more deep-seated problems. Additional remedies can be added to the treatment bottle if further symptoms present themselves. Made-up treatment bottles should be stored in a cool place and are usable for three weeks. Rescue Remedy can be taken direct from the tincture bottle—four drops on the tongue or in a glass of water sipped during the day. You may add twenty drops to a bath. If making into a compress, use six drops to a pint of water.

You can safely take Bach Flower Remedies for as long as you feel it is necessary. They can be used alone or to complement other healing methods, both conventional and holistic.

CASE HISTORIES

The case history examples given below are for general guidance. One remedy, Walnut (type and mood) belonging to the group 'over-sensitive to influences and ideas' is invaluable in menopausal difficulties, as it seeks to ease the attendant suffering during transitional stages in life.

DIANE

At forty-eight and newly divorced, Diane had returned to office work full time, after a long break at home with her two girls aged eighteen and eight.

Diane's home life had not been happy. She was an only child whose mother had criticised and nagged her and she had grown to become a fearful, timid, unhappy woman, eager to escape into the arms of the first man who would marry her. Any hopes of happiness were dashed as a result of her husband's constant drinking, their shortage of money and his aggressive criticism of her interest in holistic therapies and Friends of the Earth. Diane was almost relieved when she was able to divorce him on the grounds of his adultery. Without the support of her friends, she said, she would not have made it through the acrimonious battles over the children, finance and property, but she remained apprehensive about what might lie ahead in the world of independence, employment and childminders.

Although a natural administrator, Diane found herself fearful and dismayed by the introduction of new computer technology at work, lacking the confidence to develop new skills. She noticed that she would often have a hot flush when she felt panicky and under pressure. Beside the discomfort, the redness of her face and neck caused her acute embarrassment. One day when she had gone home feeling exhausted and in tears, she realised that unless she took action to recover her health and balance, her job security might be threatened. In addition, Diane's daughters were feeling upset by their mother's unhappiness.

She looked at her symptoms: hot flushes and night sweats which disturbed her sleep, fatigue, stress incontinence occurring at least once a week, weight gain, lack of concentration, forgetfulness and depression. She also examined the personality behind them: timid, fearful and invalidated.

Diane could not afford to consult an alternative practitioner at that time and decided to treat herself. Not wishing to have HRT she chose the Bach Flower remedies as her primary avenue of treatment, selecting Mimulus as her type (fearful, timid, shy) to help overcome her feelings of self-consciousness and agitation connected with the hot flushes; Larch for her lack of confidence; Walnut to help her adjust to the changes in personal and working circumstances; Gentian for the depression (known cause) and discouragement; and Olive for the fatigue.

Diane joined a self-awareness group, as she wished to work to release the deep-set patterns of fear and invalidation which continued to cause her problems. Within that group, she set up a menopause support group. Among other things, they investigated dietary needs and supplements and Diane decided to omit the foods and drink from her diet which were aggravating her hot flushes and night sweats. These were coffee, chocolate and curries. She took the herb Horsetail to assist with the problems of stress incontinence. The group also explored various relaxation techniques.

Diane discussed her problems in the office with her boss and they agreed that she should be sent on a computer course. As a result, she was better able to cope at work, her confidence grew and she began to enjoy her tasks.

The members of the support group observed the gradual change in Diane's attitude, which became lighter, more confident and in control. As her emotional and physical symptoms improved, she omitted those flower remedies which were no longer appropriate and added others where needed. She no longer has hot flushes or stress incontinence, has lost weight and feels more energetic.

JULIE

Julie was forty-nine and a grandmother when her husband of twenty-five years suddenly left her, after a series of affairs, to live with a much younger woman. This came as a great surprise to all who knew them, as she had never given any indication—even to her children—that anything was amiss.

Always cheerful, endlessly busy and willing to help others, Julie was dedicated to her family and making the home a happy, peaceful place. She avoided talking about herself, even when asked, and would swiftly change the subject. When she had been seriously ill, she had made light of the situation and was reluctant to discuss it or confide in anyone.

Julie had sensed for many years that her husband was

being unfaithful to her. She could not bring herself to confront him, as she knew she would be unable to cope with the major upheaval that such action could bring. She was never happier than when her children were around her and felt bereaved when they married and left home. Her husband's leaving shortly afterwards compounded this grief.

Disguising her feelings well, to the outside world Julie put on a brave face and appeared to be carrying on with life. What was going on inside her was another matter. She had always suffered from insomnia, but now the painful thoughts churning in her mind prevented her from sleeping more than two or three hours a night. She also felt very insecure and deeply depressed. Her situation appeared hopeless and she could see no way out.

Julie's daughter knew a Bach flower remedy therapist who was also a counsellor and Julie took the big step of consulting her. She was given Agrimony as a type remedy to help her share her problems and become more optimistic about the future; Walnut to help her adjust to the new circumstances at home and release the links with her estranged husband; Star of Bethlehem for her insecurity and to ease the grief felt as a result of her children leaving home, her husband's infidelity and the shock of his leaving; and Sweet Chestnut for the hopelessness and extreme anguish. In addition, Valerian tablets were suggested for the sleeping problem and Julie was thrilled at the difference they made. She saw the Bach therapist twice a month for a year. Many issues came to the surface to be dealt with, for instance, why she could not make changes and why she valued herself so little that she had allowed herself to remain in this situation. Julie was able to release deep-set patterns of parental control and repression as a result. She became more open and confident about her new direction in life.

Julie had also recently developed physical menopausal symptoms. Her menstrual cycle had become erratic and she found regular palpitations frightening. She had a tendency to high blood pressure and had previously avoided medical treatment by taking Chinese herbs. She returned to the Chinese medicine practitioner for further help; after a few months the palpitations disappeared and the menstrual cycle regulated.

Now, at almost fifty-one, Julie is feeling very well and happy. She decided to move to a small cottage by the sea where she had some friends. She is now teaching painting to small groups at a spiritual centre and retreat.

SUZANNE

Suzanne had joined a company of city stockbrokers after leaving university and had worked her way up to a senior position. She had just had her fiftieth birthday and, although used to working under extreme pressure, had begun making some catastrophic mistakes at the office.

Having made every effort to pull herself together, Suzanne was becoming worried at the lack of improvement. She was aware that she was a highly-strung person, but had recently felt increasingly tense and irritable. She seemed to have no control over her rapidly changing moods. Suzanne felt very depressed at the thought of being fifty. Although she had chosen to be a career woman, she was now very conscious of being on her own with no children. Deep in her heart she resented this.

Suzanne had been actively involved with a religious group but was beginning to feel that it was taking too much of her energy, that she was using it as a prop and that the time had come for her to let it go.

Being a very private person, Suzanne found it difficult to explain her symptoms to her doctor. He suggested that the physical symptoms she was experiencing—tiredness, headaches and indigestion—were stress-related. They talked about the menopause and he offered her tranquillisers. He also suggested painkillers and antacid tablets.

Preferring to try natural methods first, Suzanne decided to see a Bach flower remedy therapist. The treatment started with Vervain, which was her type remedy, to help her relax; Impatiens for the irritability and tension; Schleranthus was added to help with the mood swings and confusion; Willow for the introspective depression and resentment; and Walnut for adjustment to the new phase in her life. Suzanne took up various relaxation techniques suggested by the therapist. Although it took a little while to get into, she particularly enjoyed her daily meditation.

Suzanne continued taking the Bach remedies for a year and enjoyed the involvement with the practitioner in returning her to health and balance. She was delighted to observe how much more relaxed and accepting she was. She felt she had more clarity and her attitude became quite cheerful and optimistic. She was no longer troubled by mood swings and confusion. Her work and relationships at the office also improved.

At fifty-one, Suzanne joined a meditation group where she met and formed a close, loving relationship with a widower who had two young children. They are now planning to marry and Suzanne is thrilled at the prospect of becoming a full-time mother.

CHAPTER SEVEN

Counselling

WHAT IS COUNSELLING?

Counselling can help everyone who elects to use the service. It is a self-help and personal evolvement process with the support of a trained practitioner. The counsellor uses a variety of support and communication skills to enable the client to express personal feelings and difficulties. This will be in a safe atmosphere, without judgment. Through the process, clients are able to clarify their feelings, explore possible solutions and develop within themselves the potential for increased fulfilment in their lives.

Engaging a counsellor is not a symptom of weakness, illness or failure on the part of the client. Quite the opposite, seeking counselling shows a willingness to acknowledge difficulties and courageousness in finding the means to deal with them. Making the first move is often the hardest part.

COUNSELLING AND THE MENOPAUSE

The menopause, a natural transitory process in a woman's life, can be greeted with many different attitudes, from joyful acceptance to grief and dread. It may mark the passage to a freer chapter, or be seen as the beginning of the end of feminine creativity. The passage through the menopause can be a positive or negative process, depending on individual attitudes, childhood programming, patterns of family behaviour and how much we care for ourselves.

SUITING YOUR NEEDS

It is important to feel that your counsellor has an empathy

with you and your situation. A good counsellor will help you to explore your feelings constructively and to understand, grow and effect your own changes, working at a level and speed which is right for you.

Some people are not ready or prepared to look too deeply into their lives and may use the time simply to let off steam. For others, it will be a life-changing process, if they are dissatisfied with their situation, want to change their fundamental condition and attitude to life and achieve a joyful understanding and self-empowerment. The process is individual to the needs of each person and has often been likened to building a bridge to cross a dangerous river.

CONTRACTS AND CONFIDENTIALITY

A counselling session usually lasts for one hour. A verbal contract will be made between client and counsellor as to how frequently they meet and how many sessions are planned. It is usual to hold sessions weekly, fortnightly or monthly and to agree to a block of around four to six sessions. Progress will then be reviewed and a joint decision made on the making of a further contract. Some clients may make occasional single appointments specifically for in-depth confrontational work, while for others, blocks of appointments may last weeks or months.

Ground rules should be established at the first session and a confidentiality agreement made between client and counsellor. Counsellors will themselves have supervisory sessions and may need advice on aspects of a case, but will not disclose a client's identity.

TRAINING AND EMPATHY

Counsellors may work in organisations such as Relate,

Samaritans, support groups and health centres or may work individually. All should have undergone training—ask about their training and qualifications. A recommendation from someone whose judgment you trust is a good way to find a bona fide counsellor. As with all aspects of life, there are 'horses for courses' and someone with every possible qualification may not have the personal skills and rapport to suit you. Shop around until you find someone who suits you and with whom you feel comfortable.

CHANGING YOUR LIFE

Many women cope with a string of changes and upheavals—puberty, marriage, childbirth, child-rearing, careers, caring for parents. They survive house moves, their adolescent children, divorce, disappointments and losses. Yet they can still find the menopause hitting them like a tidal wave, proving to be an overwhelmingly difficult time. The children may have left home, they may be divorced or estranged from their partners, in a rut or boring routine, feeling unwell and unsure of the future. For many women who have felt their life's purpose was to support and care for others, it can feel as if they are entering a void and desolate time, without purpose.

The physical changes may affect emotions and vice-versa, making this a time for reflection; coming to terms with the end of a phase of life and evaluating and grieving for what has passed. In reassessing, it is quite common to relive much earlier experiences—the good and the not so good. It can be a time of great uncertainty for some, especially if they lack supportive family and friends.

Counselling can help you express emotion, evaluate your situation, find new ways to tackle repeated patterns of behaviour, discover options and make choices.

Successful counselling can have the effect of improving your relationship with yourself. As one woman put it, 'My life had been like spinning plates, with only just enough time and energy to keep everything going. Then the menopause tripped me up. I was forced to re-think my whole life and eventually moved into a much improved quality.'

RECOGNITION

If you think you may benefit from professional help, draw up a written or mental list of your thoughts and feelings. If there is more wrong than right and you feel unable to break the pattern or effect changes, then counselling may be of help. Follow your own instincts. If you don't choose counselling, there are many other therapies that might appeal more.

If you feel you need professional help, then the rewards from counselling will be a reflection of how much you are committed to it. Positive growth and change require a willingness to explore, feel and deal with issues. It can be a wonderful experience, a positive re-birth, a true life change, where you discover the power of the hidden self and develop new skills, interests, strengths, approaches and friends.

CASE HISTORIES

CARRIE

'I wouldn't wish my childhood on anyone,' Carrie told her counsellor. She was the elder of two girls born to parents in their early forties who were generally lacking in life experience. Their marriage was not a happy one. The girls had to endure an unpleasant atmosphere and frequent parental rows. Father was an academic, distant, idle and into his books. Mother was unable to cope with everyday family life. Her behaviour was at times most irresponsible. She would leave the house and the children without saying where she was going, often staying out for hours. One of Carrie's earliest memories was the feeling of anxiety, not knowing where her mother was. She would lie in bed waiting for the street lights to go off, knowing that if her mother was not back it must be very late.

Their mother openly favoured Carrie's sister. She would call Carrie fat and ugly, which made her feel worthless. The sister, probably in an effort to gain some of her mother's time, would often lie and blame Carrie for things she had done herself. This would inevitably result in a beating for Carrie, something which was commonplace for her anyway. Being unable to cope with even the simple duty of shopping, Carrie's mother sent her, at the age of four, on her own, across a main road, to the local shops.

At seven, Carrie was expected to buy the whole week's shopping, bringing it home on the handlebars of her bicycle. She was also expected, from a very young age, to nurse her mother when she was ill. Although Carrie was extremely clever, her tense state made passing examinations difficult. She developed a fear of failure.

Carrie trained and worked as a teacher. She married a builder and they lived in a small-holding. Shortly after Carrie's eldest daughter was born, her mother, now widowed, arrived uninvited. She stayed nineteen years until she died, quite senile. Shortly after Carrie's second daughter was born, her husband left her for a woman who lived nearby and Carrie divorced him. During most of the time her mother was living with her, Carrie worked full time as a special needs teacher, running the small-holding and looking after her mother and lively daughters.

Carrie would often arrive home to chaos and hysteria.

Her mother was controlling, possessive and selfish. Her attitude was unpredictable and she turned the rest of the family against Carrie by telling them lies. Carrie told the counsellor she felt as though she was carrying a great weight on her back throughout this time. Although she tried to lead a normal life, have relationships and hobbies and take part in community activities, arthritis had become a problem and, by the age of thirty-five, her health had deteriorated so much that she was told she would have to spend the rest of her life in a wheelchair. After her mother died, Carrie moved house, remaining at work even though she was exhausted most of the time. An unsatisfactory relationship further drained her.

At forty-seven Carrie retired early on the grounds of ill-health. ME was diagnosed. Shortly after this, menopausal symptoms started and she had to cope with headaches, hot flushes, lack of sleep and disturbed digestion. She was depressed, exhausted and unable to function. HRT disagreed with her and she sought alternative therapies, combining homoeopathy, spinal touch therapy, healing, meditation and counselling.

Counselling helped Carrie understand her need to please everyone and accept that she was still lovable if she pleased herself and made mistakes. She took up painting and music, for which she had previously not had the time. The result, after much trial and error, is that Carrie now enjoys life on her own terms, does not rush about achieving, has enlisted the help of others, learned to say 'No' and is no longer driven by others' needs. She finished the unsatisfactory relationship and no longer feels the need to depend on a man. She is prepared to consider the possibility of a quality relationship if it should ever arise. She now likes herself, is more tranquil, has made new friends and would not turn back the clock.

CHERYL

Cheryl had always had a fear of being noticed. In fact, she made an art form of merging into the background. Her parents and brother had been killed in a bombing raid towards the end of the war. At the time Cheryl was a baby. With her home completely demolished and no relatives who were able to take her, she was raised in an orphanage until she was sixteen, then fostered.

For the next thirty years, Cheryl worked in the kitchens of a local hospital. She was respected and liked by her colleagues, who knew her as a quiet, reserved, almost subdued person, with a respect for authority. Cheryl was shy and lacked confidence, preferring to stay at home. She did not appear interested in having boyfriends or going out socially.

It came as a surprise to everyone when Cheryl, at forty-three, married a widower with two children. At first she was happy, quietly looking after her husband and his daughter, who had Down's syndrome. Her stepson of sixteen was 'difficult' and had boarded for some years at a remedial school. On the boy's return home permanently, Cheryl soon found that she could not cope with him. He was disrespectful and openly resented her presence. From raiding the larder, he progressed to stealing money and other items from the house which he would sell to buy drugs. Cheryl would often come home to find the house full of his friends who had little regard for the home furnishings.

Cheryl's stepdaughter's health began to deteriorate. She became incontinent, disruptive and difficult to manage. Cheryl's husband was not much help. He seemed to be suffering from suppressed guilt about his late wife who, he felt, had possibly died as a result of being overloaded with the stress of rearing difficult children. Cheryl, dismayed to discover that he was still carrying a torch for his dead wife, felt invalidated.

She developed gall-bladder problems, together with constriction of her chest, leading to severe breathing difficulty. Cheryl's doctor told her he thought her chest problems were stress-related. She suffered extreme embarrassment at work when she turned a beetroot colour whilst having a hot flush. A nurse friend at the hospital suggested counselling. Cheryl approached several counsellors before finding one with whom she felt comfortable. She was able to explore her deep-seated anger at the loss of her family—the bewilderment of not having close family relationships and guidance. She was able to express the anger and pain at her strict institutional upbringing, during which she had felt she had no voice or any rights.

It took two years of working through these deep-seated problems before Cheryl was able to acknowledge her individuality and previously hidden lovely nature. She traced an elderly aunt who had emigrated as a GI bride and discovered she had cousins in America. Counselling helped Cheryl value herself. She was able to put her problems into perspective. Her confidence increased, enabling her to state her requirements. At one point, she went as far as saying she would leave her husband if changes were not made. She was pleased to observe her ability to talk through concerns.

Cheryl was able to report to her doctor that she felt less tense and very much better in herself. Her relationship with her husband improved and he stopped running away from the situation with his son. The boy requested counselling, which was most helpful, and his behaviour slowly changed for the better. The arrival of a girlfriend on the scene almost turned him into a model son! The stepdaughter was taken into permanent care.

Cheryl and her husband have been able to rebuild their relationship. She expressed a desire to travel, so they bought a camper van and are now becoming quite adventurous with holidays and short breaks.

REBECCA

Rebecca was one of six children. The family were Christian Scientists. At seventeen she was extremely ill with glandular fever, which left her weak. After this, she chose to stay at home with her widowed father. She led a quiet, circumspect life, married late and had three children.

The marriage was never really happy. Rebecca had a strong personality and would never admit to being wrong or apologise. She was introspective, keeping worries and feelings under tight control and any form of emotional discussion was discouraged. Rebecca and her husband often fought like cat and dog and the relationship deteriorated to the point where they were almost living separate lives.

Menopausal symptoms started when Rebecca was forty-six. She experienced menstrual flooding and sick migraines which were so severe she had to remain in bed. Nutrition had always interested her and, being an avid reader, she studied ways in which she could help herself by making dietary changes—her symptoms then improved.

When, at this difficult time in her life, Rebecca's husband died after a series of strokes, she was beside herself with remorse. Her belief in the power of the mind to heal prompted her to consult a practitioner/counsellor within the church. As a result of her meetings with the counsellor,

Rebecca was able to address her fears that she was worthless (all her brothers and sisters had reached academic excellence and had successful careers and marriages). Also, she was able to explore her fears of being without the means to support herself. Once able to recognise her value and trust more in spiritual support, she was able to step onto her spiritual pathway. She gained an understanding of the sequence of events in her life and how to deal with them.

Her entire character changed for the better. She began to enjoy life and company. Her relationship with her children improved to the point where she was invited to accompany her son and his wife to Spain on holiday. While Rebecca was in Spain, she met a Catalonian man. She fell in love—a new experience for her. They married and now live in Spain.

CHAPTER EIGHT

Eastern Medicine

Unless we change direction, we are likely to end up where we are headed.

(Chinese proverb)

Increasingly, we learn from other cultures. In recent years, there has been a rapid rise in the popularity of Eastern medicine, with interest in its study and use continuing to grow. Major therapies such as yoga, Ayurveda, Shiatsu and Traditional Chinese Medicine, which contain a wealth of wisdom and experience, are now widely available and well established in Western society.

YOGA

WHAT IS YOGA?

Over the past twenty-five years there has been an upsurge of interest in yoga, mainly amongst women seeking relaxation and to maintain personal fitness.

Yoga was devised in India over 5000 years ago. It has eight methods, or 'limbs', including contemplation, meditation, breathing (pranayama) and curative physical postures (asanas). Fundamental to basic yoga philosophy is the existence of a vital healing energy. A network of pathways (nadis) conveys this energy around the body. The functions of the organs and systems are controlled by seven energy centres (chakras)—a theory also understood in Western healing.

Yoga sees the body, mind and breath as being interdependent. Its aim is to unify body and mind to the point where the individual attains inner peace, allowing space for the body to heal itself. As a system it can help with all aspects of mental and physical well-being. Regular practice maintains a balanced state of health.

HOW CAN YOGA HELP IN MENOPAUSE?

Hatha yoga is the name given to the type of yoga practised most in the West. It uses the natural functions of stretching and breathing. A typical session will include a short period of initial relaxation, a series of postures, breathing exercises and final relaxation. Yoga is able to help with many of the stress-related problems commonly experienced in menopause, such as anxiety, panic attacks, depression, insomnia and weight reduction, as well as a large range of physical problems.

TRYING YOGA FOR YOURSELF

You do not need to have a deep religious or spiritual commitment in order to practise yoga, but many people find it brings about self-realisation and a positive change in attitudes. Numerous books and videos are available for beginners, which can be useful, but the best way to learn is to join a class, especially if you wish to use yoga for therapeutic purposes. There are various schools of yoga and it is advisable to enquire about the type being taught before deciding on a class, for example whether the routine is of a more physical nature or whether the emphasis is on gentle postures, breathing and meditation. You may have to shop around for a teacher and class that suits you.

In the main, yoga classes are an inexpensive, sociable and supportive experience. Students are encouraged to proceed at their own pace, within their own boundaries. Some teachers are available for private consultation and tuition.

Setting aside half-an-hour or so each day for yoga practice at home is a very beneficial way of switching off and recharging your batteries. A yoga session should leave you feeling uplifted, relaxed and more in touch with your inner world.

AYURVEDA
WHAT IS AYURVEDA?

Two Sanskrit words are joined to form the word Ayurveda: *ayur*, meaning 'knowledge' or 'knowing' and *veda*, meaning 'life'. Ayurveda is a comprehensive natural healing system which originated in India at least 5000 years ago. It is holistic in that it does not separate the physical/psychological/ emotional from the cause or treatment of people or diseases. Having its roots in yoga, it has a strong spiritual and philosophical foundation. In ancient times, Ayurveda included a sophisticated, complete medical system with branches of surgery and psychiatry. It was considered a route to spiritual enlightenment. Today, although it can be used as a foundation for spiritual practices, Ayurveda centres on the use of herbs and diet in a practical self-help way, and on treating illness once created.

Some of the major healing systems throughout the world have been strongly influenced by Ayurveda, including the Chinese element system, Middle Eastern and Greek medicine. The associations with Ayurveda continue into modern times, with several of its methods now being incorporated into naturopathy. Ayurveda is a way of life to the majority of the large Asian community in Britain. During the last few years, we have embraced their food and are now also beginning to use their simple and holistic way of healing.

One of the fundamental principles of Ayurveda is that the

energy of life is expressed through three 'doshas', known as Vata, Pitta and Kapha. People are a mixture of the doshas, but usually one is considered to be dominant and another secondary.

How can Ayurveda Help in Menopause?

In Ayurveda, problems in menopause relate to deficiency and change. The dosha of Vatu governs change and also relates to depletion and stress. Menopause is therefore a Vata related condition, but it can also be Kapha or Pitta.

Ayurvedic methods can help in the treatment and prevention of all menopausal conditions. Practitioners use several traditional holistic methods of diagnosis to assess an individual's constitution and condition. However, it is quite possible to use Ayurveda on a self-help basis. The Ayurvedic Trading Company mentioned in Useful Addresses provides information and a catalogue of products. The Ayurvedic advisor for this book recommends aloe vera juice as one of the most useful remedies for menopausal complaints.

Shiatsu

What is Shiatsu?

Shiatsu, a word of Japanese origin meaning 'finger pressure', is a practical bodywork therapy based on pressure, touch and stretching—healing techniques which have been used throughout the world for thousands of years. Developed from an ancient Japanese healing art of hand and foot massage, Shiatsu emerged as an independent holistic healing therapy in the early part of the twentieth century.

Shiatsu and acupressure have in common the use of applied pressure on the hundreds of pressure points found along the body's meridians and elsewhere. The Shiatsu techniques tend to be more versatile, using the fingers, thumbs, palms, fists, elbows, knees and feet to stimulate or calm the pressure points to release tension and blockages. The approach to Shiatsu varies widely, with different methods and styles being used. Some practitioners adopt a more physical approach, others might prefer to work more gently.

HOW CAN SHIATSU HELP IN MENOPAUSE?

The healthy body is a self-regulating mechanism, working constantly to achieve a state of dynamic balance—in body, mind and spirit. Menopause is a natural process, not intended to cause suffering. If the body is in dynamic balance, then the passage is made easier. Perhaps the main obstacle to achieving this balance is the individual's reaction to stress. The supportive body contact techniques used in Shiatsu make them particularly appealing to women as a therapy, affording a simple but effective way of relaxing, releasing tension and managing stress. Shiatsu is based on a process termed 'relax, release and let go', but it works at all levels to intrinsically balance the body's flow of energy. The aim is to bring the individual to a state of relaxation and stillness of body and mind in which the process of healing and personal transformation can begin.

Because Shiatsu is based on relaxation and stress release, it can help a wide range of health problems and holds many benefits for women in preventative and curative health care. It can help to:
- calm the nervous system
- lower the blood pressure
- improve the cardiovascular system and lymphatic flow
- balance the hormonal system

- strengthen the digestive system
- strengthen the immune system
- improve general flexibility, health and vitality
- help to slow the 'ageing' or maturation process
- improve the condition of the skin and hair
- increase libido
- alleviate aches and pains
- improve muscle tone
- strengthen the skeletal system
- re-create a balanced sleep pattern.

SHIATSU TREATMENT

Shiatsu can be studied on a self-help basis, to share with a friend or partner and in this way can be very rewarding. But for maximum benefit, it is preferable to experience Shiatsu in the hands of a trained registered practitioner who is able to intuitively locate the pressure points and search out the deeper causes of tension.

A Shiatsu session with a registered practitioner will last about an hour. It should take place in a warm, quiet environment, normally at floor level on a mat or blanket. For the pressure, stretching and manipulative techniques to have any real effect, the body and mind must feel relaxed, so treatment should begin with a pleasurable, supportive relaxation routine. This is done in combination with the breath—keeping the mouth slightly open, breathing in through the nose and out through the mouth. The body cannot relax sufficiently if the jaw is tight, so this kind of breathing, which is also used to assist the release process, is continued throughout the session.

The whole body is involved in the treatment. Within the recipient's comfort zone, the use of finger and thumb pressure, palming, rocking movements, gentle manipulation, kneading and stretching techniques can be expected. Shiatsu is also a therapy of communication, trust, feedback and support. During treatment, many emotions and bodily sensations may be experienced. Feelings of deep relaxation, happiness and peace are commonly reported, as are the sensations of heat and sometimes 'positive pain', when the points are being worked. All are signs that the body is making adjustments in order to reach a more dynamically balanced state.

Self-help measures can be continued at home, for which the practitioner may offer healthier lifestyle suggestions, including relaxation and breathing techniques, remedial exercises and dietary recommendations.

TRADITIONAL CHINESE MEDICINE
WHAT IS TRADITIONAL CHINESE MEDICINE?

The history of traditional Chinese medicine (TCM) can be dated back to 2800 BC, when the supreme leader, Shen Nong (the Divine Farmer), first started using herbs to treat his citizens. It is said that he discovered the medicinal use of about one hundred plants after tasting them all himself. About 150 years later, the Yellow Emperor, a successor of the Divine Farmer, developed the therapeutic needling technique of acupuncture and the two methods joined to form one system of medicine.

Today, the TCM system includes herbal medicine, acupuncture, acupressure, massage, Tai Ji Quan (T'ai-chi) and Qi Gong exercises and dietary therapy. A patient visiting a TCM practitioner will not only be given herbal remedies and/or acupuncture, but will also receive advice on exercise and diet that may enhance the effectiveness of the treatment.

For thousands of years, TCM practitioners have believed that diseases can be prevented just as effectively as they can be treated. For example, regular head massage can help to reduce the intensity of the pain of a headache or completely prevent its return. Doing regular exercises like T'ai-chi or Qi Gong can improve the circulation and strengthen the immune system, helping to combat diseases.

CHOOSING A PRACTITIONER

Although many Westerners are now practising TCM, it is likely that you will be treated by a Chinese practitioner, maybe with an interpreter present. It is fair to say that if a combination of acupuncture and herbs is given, it can make the treatment a little expensive. Acupuncture/acupressure is widely available as a treatment on its own.

HOW DOES TCM VIEW YOUR BODY?
(a) Yin and Yang

During its formation and in the early years, TCM was greatly influenced by the philosophy of Yin and Yang, which holds that Yin and Yang are two forces existing in the cosmos. They are opposite to each other, and yet mutually dependent.

Things that are watery, moist, still, cold, slow, descending, etc. pertain to Yin. Things that are fiery, dry, active, hot, fast, ascending etc. pertain to Yang. The perfect balance of these two forces within your body allows you to benefit from good health. If one of the forces is depleted, the other will also be affected.

When Yin is deficient, symptoms like hot flushes, night sweats, thirst, restlessness and insomnia may be experienced. If, on the other hand, Yang is deficient, symptoms such as chills, cold hands and feet, tiredness, swollen ankles and increased urination may occur. Once the balance between

Yin and Yang is restored, these symptoms will disappear or improve.

(b) Qi

Qi is regarded as the vital energy and life force found everywhere in the body. It dominates the body's growth and development, promotes blood circulation, regulates body temperature and fights disease. When Qi is plentiful, physical and emotional activity is buoyant. If Qi becomes weak or stagnated, symptoms like slow growth, poor immunity, slow healing process and muscle and joint pains may occur.

The passages along which Qi travels are called meridians. They connect the body surface to the internal organs. Thus, any changes inside the body will manifest on the surface. During an acupuncture treatment, fine needles are used to stimulate some Qi points located on the surface meridian.

In TCM, various emotions are linked to different organs: joy is related to the heart, anger and frustration to the liver, and pensiveness and worry to the spleen. Sadness is associated with the lungs.

HOW DOES TCM EXPLAIN MENOPAUSE?

In TCM, the physiological activities in women are controlled by Tian Kui, which is a type of female essence stored inside the kidneys. It directs that female physiological development follows a seven-year cycle. So at the age of fourteen, menstruation begins, her womb starts to develop and she becomes fertile. When she reaches twenty-one, her female organs are fully developed and therefore it is the best time to bear children. When she is about forty-nine years of age, Tian Kui deteriorates; her periods gradually stop and she is no longer able to conceive.

Apart from menstrual and fertility changes, various physical and emotional symptoms may also be seen during menopause. Some common ones are fatigue, brittle bones and nails, loose teeth, soreness of the lower back and knees, puffy eyes, swollen ankles, poor memory, dry eyes, thrush, low or raised libido, mood swings and lack of willpower and confidence. These symptoms can be related mainly to the kidneys, which are responsible for the strength of the bones and teeth, proper memory, transporting fluids and libido. Often, using acupuncture or herbs to tone the kidneys can achieve a desirable healing effect.

According to whether the kidney deficiency is yin or yang, certain everyday foods might be recommended to support treatment. These include sesame seeds, walnuts, peanuts, black beans, some seafoods, asparagus, lychees and lamb. Herbal tinctures may be given to drink.

How do TCM Practitioners Treat Menopause?

Commonly-used treatments in TCM include acupuncture, acupressure, Chinese herbal medicine, dietary therapy and Qi exercises. Two people may have similar symptoms, but receive quite different treatment. This is because TCM takes into account not only the symptoms but a person's age, constitution, lifestyle and emotional state. The following treatments can be used alone or in combination. In expert hands, every treatment should be tailor-made to suit the individual's condition. Treatment may be adjusted from time to time during a course.

Acupuncture

Most of us dislike the idea of injections. Therefore, it is very easy to jump to the conclusion that the size of an acupuncture needle is similar to that of a syringe needle, whereas in fact, it is not that much thicker than a single hair.

The needles are used to stimulate specific points on the surface meridians. The purpose is to regulate the volume and flow of Qi inside channels and organs. Sometimes, an acupuncturist, after inserting a needle, will put a short herbal stick made from the herb mugwort on the handle of the needle and burn it. This supplementary treatment is called moxibustion and is very effective for cold, deficiency and chronic conditions.

For acute problems, it is normally advisable to have treatment sessions close to each other over a short period of time, for example, every two to three days for a course of ten treatments. When the condition is chronic, the patient is likely to be asked to attend treatment weekly over a longer period. When the situation improves, the frequency of treatment will be reduced. In most cases, people feel very relaxed after an acupuncture session and will be asked not to do strenuous exercise after the treatment.

Acupressure
Many TCM practitioners use acupressure as a method of treatment, often combining it with massage. Acupressure works in much the same way as acupuncture, but instead of needles, finger pressure is used to stimulate the points.

Many conditions benefit from acupressure. It is particularly useful, on its own or with acupuncuture, when treating pain in the lower abdomen and back and in problems of the muscular skeletal system. Muscular spasms are a good case where it is often easier to use acupressure.

SELF HELP USING ACUPRESSURE

It is always useful to remember some simple methods of treating yourself when your practitioner is not available. Here are several acupressure points you can use to relieve some of the symptoms you may experience.

For insomnia, anxiety, panic attacks, palpitations:
Use Shen Meng, a point on the heart meridian and Nei Guan, a point on the pericardium meridian. Press with your thumb until you get a sore sensation on the points, then gently massage on each point on both hands for five minutes. Massage two to three times a day, or when you feel you are under stress. For insomnia, massage once more 15-30 minutes before going to bed.

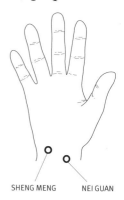

SHENG MENG   NEI GUAN

For headaches and dizziness: Use Feng Chi on the gallbladder meridian and Tai Chong on the liver meridian. Press with your thumb and massage for five

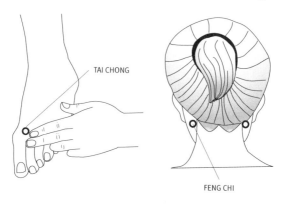

TAI CHONG

FENG CHI

minutes on each point on both sides. Massage two or three times a day, also before or during an attack.

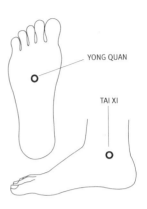

For hot flushes and night sweats: Use Yong Quan and Tai Xi on the kidney meridian. Follow the same instructions as for headaches and dizziness.

Chinese Herbal Medicine

There are about 300 herbs which are commonly used. After a consultation, a herbalist will usually prescribe ten to fifteen dried herbs, which are normally given to the patient in bags; the number of these will vary according to the individual's condition. The patient will be asked to make an infusion out of these herbs and drink it daily. For those who are not able to find time to make their own herbal teas, concentrated herbal powders, capsules, tinctures and pills can be used as alternatives. However, most Chinese herbalists believe that the best results come from drinking the herbal infusions, despite their unique taste. A course of herbal treatment will entail taking the herbs daily until the condition improves.

Advice on Diet and Exercise

In addition to acupuncture or herbal medicine, advice on dietary habits is often given by practitioners. It is believed that eating the right food, in the right amounts and at regular times, is important for good health. For example, those who suffer from painful and swollen joints are often advised to eat less greasy, raw and cold-natured food. Those who find it difficult to get to sleep or have disturbed sleep should try to avoid hot, spicy food.

Like herbal medicines, foods have their own qualities, such as cold, hot, drying, moisturising, etc. Avoiding or eating more of certain foods can help to change the constitution of the body.

Some practitioners also recommend exercises like T'ai-chi and Qi Gong. These exercises have been used by Chinese people for thousands of years. Most Chinese, whatever their age, still keep up the habit of getting up early in the morning to exercise in a park or an open space. These exercises are effective in promoting Qi and blood circulation and general relaxation. Some of the more simple, slow movements are often used in conjunction with breathing techniques. After practising for a short while, many people find they feel more relaxed and confident in themselves and that there is an improvement in their physical well-being.

SELF-HELP USING CHINESE HERBAL MEDICINE

The ways in which a Western herbalist and a TCM practitioner work, and the herbs they use, are very different. Chinese herbs are very effective in creating hormonal harmony and balance according to the principles of TCM, and will act better if the individual is treated constitutionally (with all the underlying deficiencies and imbalances being taken into account). We do not have the professional knowledge to prescribe Chinese herbs successfully for ourselves; it is therefore wiser and safer to have a consultation with a TCM practitioner.

Self-help with Chinese herbs should be approached only on a simple level. Among herbs which nourish and replenish kidney essence and regulate hormonal balance are Peony

Root, Cornus, Dioscorea and cooked Rehmannia. If used properly, they can safely be taken on a regular basis.

CASE HISTORIES
CINDY

Cindy, aged forty-seven, had been living with her two children since her divorce ten years previously. For the last eighteen months, her periods had been irregular and she had been having upwards of ten hot flushes a day.

Night sweats would greatly disturb her sleep, leaving her feeling exhausted and irritable. Her relationship with the children had become very tense. She was also experiencing frequent headaches, pain and swelling in the joints and had gained one and a half stones in a year. There was not much fun in Cindy's life; she had little time to herself and felt her emotional needs were not being met. She had not had a relationship for two years and much of her time was spent looking after her widowed mother, who was a difficult and demanding woman. Cindy felt drained and lonely and was finding it difficult to cope.

Cindy had benefited from TCM in the past and decided to return to the practitioner. At her first consultation, she was diagnosed as 'uprising liver yang with underlying liver and kidney deficiency'. Her tongue was red at the tip, with teethmarks, suggesting kidney deficiency with heat in the heart. Her pulse was wiry and thin, suggesting liver yang rising and yin deficiency. She was prescribed acupuncture treatment and Chinese herbs to be boiled up at home. Acupuncture points on the liver, kidney and heart meridians were selected and needled. (They are used to subdue the liver yang, replenish the yin and calm the mind.) She was asked to have the treatment once a week for ten sessions.

After the first treatment, Cindy noticed that her sleep was less disturbed and she felt more relaxed. She took the herbal infusions every day. The herbs prescribed included Tian Ma (gastrodia tuber), Gou Teng (uncaria stem), Sang Ji Shen (mulberry mistletoe), Shu Di Huang (prepared rheumania), Gou Qi Zi (wolfberry) and Wu Wei Zi (schizandra fruit). Four weeks later, the night sweats had almost subsided and she was having only two to four hot flushes a day.

Encouraged by the improvements, Cindy continued to have both treatments for four more months. During that period, different acupuncture points and herbs were used, according to her changing condition. Menstruation is now tailing off. Cindy's joint pain and swelling is much better. She feels more energetic and confident in herself.

Maintenance treatment continues on a monthly basis, as Cindy finds this helps her to lose weight. Her personal circumstances have taken a turn for the better—she has recently started a relationship and fallen in love. Her work direction has become more fulfilling—she is doing some part-time work as a Reiki practitioner.

JASMINE

Jasmine, a forty-nine-year-old teacher in a college, is happily married and lives with her husband and two children. She first consulted a TCM practitioner two and a half years ago complaining that, although her periods were regular, they had become very heavy over the last nine months. It had been medically established that Jasmine did not have fibroids or any other underlying condition to cause the excessive bleeding. As she was becoming anaemic, an iron supplement was given and a hysterectomy was suggested.

Other symptoms were light-headedness, palpitations and

loss of clarity, especially when under a great deal of stress. She was finding it difficult to concentrate on her work, which was becoming increasingly demanding as a result of extra paperwork. She was also having a few hot flushes and night sweats. In addition, Jasmine was concerned about pain in her left hip which she had had for about a year, following a fall. The pain was becoming more frequent and was worse if she had been standing a lot. It was taking her longer to walk to the bus station. Because her mother had recently had a hip replacement operation, Jasmine was worried that she might need one too if the pain became unbearable. Although she is a very confident person, the possibility distressed her.

Chinese medicine was recommended by friends and, being willing to try anything to get better, Jasmine went to see a practitioner. After the consultation, she was diagnosed as having 'heart and spleen deficiency with depleted kidney essence'. A six-month programme of treatment was arranged. Both acupuncture and Chinese herbs were used.

During the acupuncture treatment, moxa sticks were also used, together with some points on the spleen and kidney meridians. This was to help boost the Qi to stop the bleeding, as well as to strengthen the bones and joints. The joint pain improved immediately after just one session. At the same time, Jasmine took herbal powders every day as she didn't have enough time to boil the herbs. Herbs used included Dang Gui (angelica root), Bai Zhu (white atractylodes tuber), Dang Shen (codonopsis root), Qian Cao (madder root) and Mu dan Pi (tree peony bark). Three months later, the bleeding had decreased considerably and Jasmine had regained her vitality. Her periods have now almost finished. She still attends for treatment for her hip. Otherwise she is feeling very well and thinking of taking up T'ai-chi to help improve her general health.

CHAPTER NINE

Healing

'Love makes the world go round' ..., a phrase often used lightly but, in terms of healing, it is recognised that a universal force of love connects and supports everything on our living planet.

One of the oldest therapies known to humankind, healing, or the laying on of hands, is seen in its simplest form in the love that a mother has for her child, soothing by touch and loving thoughts and words. Embracing and projecting acceptance, unconditional love and compassion, healers seek to tap into and use this unseen source of energy for the benefit of those in need and seeking help.

Helping a wide range of physical, emotional and psychological problems, healing works well with all methods of therapy or it can stand alone. It is gentle and produces no side-effects. By raising the deeper levels of awareness, inner blocks which have prevented good health can be released, allowing the body to re-balance and return to peace, harmony and wholeness. Also, where necessary, healing can calm a troubled spirit and ease the passage into the next world.

A BRIEF HISTORY OF HEALING

We are all healers, in that we possess the ability to have a positive healing influence on ourselves, others and the world around us by using the power of touch and thought. This innate ability and the recognition of a positive unseen force has always been part of our existence. History provides us with a wealth of evidence in support of this. Healing philosophy is part of every ancient religion. We know that hands-on healing was included in the spiritual practices of the temple priests in the ancient Egyptian civilisation. The Bible tells us of miracles, healing acts and the wondrous works of Jesus—the healing tradition was an important part of the early Christian church. Healing systems still continue in tribal cultures, who have always relied on their shamans, medicine men and witch doctors for the performance of rituals to prevent and heal illness.

This century, the amazing healing work of the late British spiritualist Harry Edwards has done much to promote a positive image of healing, helping many to recognise their true spiritual nature. Nowadays, there are healing ministries in both the Catholic and Anglican churches and many doctors have invited healers to work in their practices, with excellent results. Recently, healing has received favourable publicity in the media, with television demonstrations as to its efficacy and reports of encouraging results from research. Public satisfaction and support has increased to the point where healing is now accepted in all areas of the community as an effective therapy in preventative and curative healthcare.

HOW CAN HEALING HELP IN MENOPAUSE?

Healing is extremely effective and supportive when used during times of transition. It can help to relieve all the physical symptoms of menopause and, as it is a particularly relaxing therapy, it is also of great use where emotional and stress-related issues are involved.

The chemical and hormonal changes which take place in a woman's body during menopause can give rise to a state of flux. Many women at this time become extremely sensitive, both in their bodies and in their awareness. The therapy of healing also works with the more subtle energies and can successfully help when heightened sensitivity is a problem.

Menopause can be a very trying time for many women. It may prompt some to take a look at their lives—past, present and future—with a view to easing feelings of isolation, making changes and moving on. Healing can help in finding the quiet, inner space where solutions to problems and realisation of personal power can be found.

GIVING AND RECEIVING

Healers' views on the way healing works may differ according to their religious convictions and other beliefs, but all will agree that an exchange of energy takes place between healer and patient. The healer acts as a channel for healing energies to pass through and connect with the self-healing mechanism of the patient. The healer's prime responsibility is to remain an emotionally clear channel, giving the healing energies free passage. Many healers are aware of an invisible field or aura surrounding the body and energy centres within it (this is also part of the basic philosophy of many Eastern healing techniques.) They work to bring these centres into balance. Although healers will have their own routine, all work with their hands lightly touching and at a short distance from the body.

HEALER TRAINING

Although we all possess the gift of healing, some of us are strongly motivated to develop and use it for the benefit of others. With a healer membership in excess of 7000—working both individually and in groups and centres—the

National Federation of Spiritual Healers (NFSH) is the largest healing organisation in Britain. It has a full programme of basic healer development courses which are available throughout the country. Accreditation as an NFSH healer requires more than learning a 'hands-on' healing routine. Among the subjects covered in the training syllabus are: self-healing and the responsibility of being a healer; spiritual attunement in relation to healing; meditation; creative visualisation; relaxation and stress management; breath and breathing; the nature of disease; the energy centres; our invisible bodies; distant healing; colour, sound and movement; childhood influences on personal balance; seeking the message of disease; healing to ease death and dying. Most healers will also have undertaken some form of counselling training.

Most healers who belong to healing organisations which are members of the Confederation of Healing Organisations are non-denominational. They are bound by a strict code of conduct and are not permitted to make any diagnosis or prognosis. A few healers give their services free, others make a set charge or accept donations. If you are unable to find a local healer, the NFSH will be happy to provide you with the names of one or two healers in your area (see Useful Addresses). The example of a healing session below is in accordance with NFSH guidelines.

A HEALING SESSION

When choosing a healer, look for one with whom you have a feeling of rapport. The healing environment should be relaxing, comfortable and supportive, as an emotional release of pent-up stress can often take place. Patients normally sit down to receive healing, but sometimes lying down is more appropriate. After telling the healer how you wish to be helped, and perhaps a short informal discussion, you will be invited to close your eyes and relax. Receiving healing is an ideal opportunity to rest the mind. Some patients may prefer to do their own meditation or visualisation; otherwise the Buddhist practice of watching the breath referred to in Chapter 12 Meditation is a good exercise. Alternatively, you may prefer simply to imagine a scene where you feel peaceful and happy. Unwanted thoughts invariably pass through the mind—acknowledge these and let them go, before returning to your quiet state.

Healing will normally start with the healer standing behind you for a few minutes with their hands on your shoulders, in order to attune to the universal energy force and enter into a short mental routine of prayer/affirmation. This may include a request that the healer and patient are grounded and protected in love and light; that the patient is brought into balance and harmony and made whole according to divine will; trusting that the outcome will be to the patient's highest good.

The healer will normally begin with their hands a short distance from your head and then, with particular emphasis on the energy centres, work slowly down the body to your feet. Extra attention will be paid to areas of difficulty or where the healer intuitively feels there is a need. The hands, ankles and feet are normally held for a short time. The healer will return to your shoulders, mentally closing down and releasing you. You are then gently told to open your eyes when you are ready.

The healing act takes twenty to thirty minutes. Most patients comment on how relaxed they feel afterwards. Each healing experience, for patient and healer, is different.

Warmth, coolness, tingling and other sensations are often felt. The release of unwanted emotions by way of gentle weeping sometimes occurs during a healing. Here are some comments which I, as a healer, have personally noted:

'I saw deep blue and purple.'
'The pain worsened for a few seconds and then went away.'
'I feel so relaxed and peaceful.'
'I could smell the herb Rosemary.'
'I never realised how much my father loved me.'
'I felt my spine clicking into place.'

The benefits of healing are not always immediately obvious. They are often seen in the way people begin to help themselves by letting go of old attitudes and patterns of behaviour and making positive changes—leading to an improvement in health and quality of life.

ABSENT HEALING

It is not necessary for the person needing healing to be present for healing to be given. It can be sent 'absently' by thought. Many healing and meditation groups hold lists for this purpose. Permission does not have to be obtained for absent healing to be sent, as we can all choose on an unseen level whether or not to accept what is offered.

SELF-HELP

Self-healing is a simple route to personal growth and better health. You might like to try a short exercise to sense your own energy:

Rub the palms of your hands together for a few seconds;

clap your hands a few times, then hold them about twenty inches apart and very slowly draw them together. Your hands are passing through your own energy field. Every few inches or so you will feel a subtle resistance. This marks the 'layers' of your invisible body or aura.

Some people can see the human aura in the form of colours. Most of us can see the etheric layer around ourselves and others:

Try holding up your hands twenty inches or so away from your body, fingers slightly apart, with a white wall in the background. The room lighting should not be bright. Then, with a relaxed gaze, look 'through' your fingers for a few seconds. You will see a bluish-grey outline around your fingers; this is your etheric body.

Many people say they just *cannot* visualise. But we do it all the time! For example, what happens when you think of something delicious to eat? Your mouth waters.

Try this simple visualisation:

Sit quietly, close your eyes and imagine you are at a vegetable stall buying lemons. Concentrate on the lemons—observe their bright yellow colour and the texture of their skins. The stall holder selects a lemon and cuts it in half, inviting you to take a bite. You do … Ugh! Yes you *can* visualise!

Now that you have established better contact with yourself, you might like to try a little personal 'hands-on' healing in using these simple five-minute exercises.

(a) Hold your hand/s over an area of your body where you have a problem. Visualise blue healing light travelling down your arm through your hand/s into the area and it returning to health.

(b) Sit down and breathe deeply for a minute or two. Hold your hands a few inches apart. Imagine golden energy coming up through your feet—through your body and into your hands—to form a ball. Hold the ball, take it above your head, then, using it to cleanse and heal, take it to the parts of your body which are tense and painful.

If appropriate, healers will give their patients ideas for self-help work at home. They might suggest particular visualisations and affirmations to help turn around a negative situation or to release unwanted, deeply-held emotions. A particularly powerful affirmation you may like to try is:

I am now willingly releasing, with forgiveness and thankfulness, everything that I do not need, and ask that it releases me.

Other positive self-help measures by means of relaxation, breathing, visualisation, affirmations and meditation are included in the Relaxation and Meditation chapters of this book.

CASE HISTORIES
JENNY
Jenny was fifty-one. Since leaving school, she had looked after her severely disabled, widowed mother who was now senile

and had recently been admitted to a Local Authority home. The mother had been very demanding and controlling, not appearing to appreciate Jenny's dedication to caring for her.

Jenny had once had a boyfriend, but her mother had discouraged the relationship. He eventually married someone else. Jenny never became involved with another man and felt deep sadness at her lost opportunity.

When she was made redundant from a part-time clerical job in a bank, just before her mother was taken into care, Jenny felt devastated. She did not qualify for a redundancy payment and was now finding it difficult to manage on State Benefit. She attended several job interviews, but was not offered employment and was beginning to feel she was over-the-hill as far as work was concerned.

Jenny felt very depressed and lonely. There was no-one to turn to. She worried that the confusion, forgetfulness and irrational thoughts she was experiencing were signs that she would develop the same problems as her mother. She could not understand why she felt so tired when she had less work to do. Her general practitioner could find nothing wrong with Jenny's back, which ached nearly all the time. In addition, she had developed pains in her elbows and wrists and her skin had become very dry.

Jenny's mother had benefited from healing given by a healer who visited her residential care home. Jenny decided to request healing for herself at a nearby NFSH Healing Centre, where she could pay by donation.

On one occasion, the healer suggested she try a visualisation exercise of sitting down and having a dialogue with her mother in which they could both communicate their thoughts and feelings. In this way, Jenny was able to express pent-up feelings of resentment and unhappiness.

After completing the exercise to her satisfaction, Jenny exclaimed that her backache had gone. There has been no recurrence.

Jenny had eight appointments at the Healing Centre and was delighted to observe the improvements to her health. Her thoughts became calmer and she felt much more together. She loved the relaxed feeling the healing gave her. Each healing experience was different—sometimes she would have a gentle, tearful release, and on other occasions she sat back and enjoyed the beautiful colours which came flooding through her mind.

Jenny started to attend the Centre's weekly meditation and healing workshop. On applying to take a basic healing course, she was offered a bursary place. Jenny made new friends, found much support at the Centre and began to enjoy a social life. An aromatherapist friend suggested some oils for her joint pains and dry skin and after three months these symptoms disappeared.

Jenny stopped worrying about obtaining employment and she decided to use her increased free time to rest. She started a basic book-keeping course at a college of further education and was delighted to discover this was free because she was in receipt of State Benefit.

A year on, Jenny has gone from strength to strength, feels in control of her life and is now giving healing herself as a probationer healer.

SANDRA

Sandra had been born and bred in the country and was married to a farm worker. Her two sons had left home and worked in the local cheese factory. Sandra was very involved in helping look after her four grandchildren.

For the last twenty years, Sandra had worked at a nearby farm, seven days a week, assisting at morning and afternoon milking. Her wages were low, the work often hard, but Sandra enjoyed it and loved the animals. Sandra and her husband had never ventured far from their village and rarely took a holiday.

At forty-seven, she was alarmed at the changes in her menstrual cycle and the general state of her health. Her periods had become very heavy and she was feeling exhausted. Her breasts were sore. Sandra did a lot of walking as she and her husband did not possess a car. She was finding it increasingly difficult to get about, because her legs ached and were also swollen.

After having to be taken home during milking one day because of severe menstrual flooding, Sandra went to see her doctor. She was normally a sturdy, healthy person. In fact, she had only ever taken the odd painkiller and cough mixture. The doctor gave Sandra a thorough examination and found nothing wrong. Being aware of her aversion to drugs, he suggested homoeopathy, which he was also practising under the NHS. Sandra felt this would suit her.

Sandra was also friendly with a local healer from whom she requested healing. They had a regular appointment every week for six months, the sessions taking about an hour. Sandra slowly began to feel better. She often remarked after a healing session that she felt as though she had just had a night's sleep. Sandra also wished to take something herbal. Her local wholefood store suggested Borage juice, which helps regulate hormonal balance and is very useful at the time of menopause.

Sandra is now almost forty-nine and feels as though she has had a new lease of life. She has given up her job and is helping out at an old people's home. She particularly enjoys accompanying them on outings. Following a small win on the National Lottery, she is now planning a holiday in Spain.

ANNE

Anne, at forty-nine, had been a single parent for sixteen years. She worked part-time in a travel agent and her income was supplemented by State Benefit. However, it was a struggle to pay the mortgage and bills. She and her son led a quiet life. Money being short, leisure activities and holidays were thin on the ground.

Anne took a keen interest in the activities of Greenpeace. She was dismayed to learn her son had chosen to join the Army rather than go on to further education at college. The boy had been extremely difficult to handle all through puberty. On one occasion when Anne had been trying to discuss his aggressive behaviour with him, he told her that he was very angry that his father had left him when he was eleven months old to work abroad. This dredged up Anne's suppressed feelings of resentment and anger that she had reared the boy single-handed with poor financial and no emotional support.

Beside herself with anguish at the thought of her son leaving home, Anne was also worried that she might not be able to find full-time employment when her entitlement to State Benefit ceased. She felt irritable, had angry outbursts and frequently burst into tears.

Anne had experienced a short menstrual cycle since her son was born and consulted her general practitioner when the bleeding became excessive, leaving her feeling exhausted most of the time. She was told she had a large fibroid in her womb and surgery was recommended. Anne felt upset and frightened. She did not wish to have surgery.

Anne accepted an offer of healing from a healer friend. For the first month, Anne received healing twice a week. With the fibroid and menstrual problems in mind, the healer recommended a macrobiotic dietary practitioner and Anne followed this up. She was placed on a supervised diet and slowly the fibroid began to shrink to the point where, after a year, an operation was unnecessary. Anne was thrilled when her menstrual cycle lengthened and the blood flow became normal. A short course of Chinese herbs helped build her up and the exhaustion went. In fact she felt better than she had when she was thirty!

The healing continued all through this period, reducing to once a week, then twice a month. The healer encouraged Anne to so some work on acceptance, forgiveness and release and the feelings of anger and resentment towards her ex-husband abated.

Anne detected a definite shift in her attitude and reported to the healer that she felt much more cheerful, calm, in control of her life and less worried about the future. Her relationship with her son improved to the point where they were able to talk problems through and greater cooperation developed between them. He signed up to the Army for three years and was accepted on an engineering course. His experience away from home gave him a greater maturity and he had more respect for his mother. Anne's physical symptoms did not return and she continued to enjoy a better quality of life.

CHAPTER TEN

Herbal Medicine

WHAT ARE HERBS?

Herbs can be defined as any plants, including flowers and trees, which can be used medicinally or in the preparation of food. Many of these plants are familiar to us and include:

- wild flowers—Dandelion, Chamomile, Comfrey
- garden herbs—Garlic, Rosemary, Sage
- garden plants—Marigold, Cabbage, Oats, Celery
- trees—Cinnamon, Hawthorn, Witch Hazel.

In Britain, herbalists often use a mixture of native and European herbs. Increasing use is being made of plants from further afield, such as Echinacea, Black and Blue Cohosh and False Unicorn Root, all originally used by the North American Indians. Mexican Wild Yam, Ginseng and other plants from the Far East are also used.

WHAT IS HERBAL MEDICINE?

Herbal medicine is a natural, safe and unhurried method of healing using the curative properties of plants. Without producing side-effects or withdrawal symptoms, it can effectively stand alone as a system in its own right or be used alongside conventional medicine. Supported by British common law and the World Health Organisation, herbal medicine is the major form of treatment worldwide.

Herbal medicine can treat a large number of problems, from acute and everyday ailments to deep-set and serious illness. Remedies can be given internally or externally. Most prescriptions are taken in the form of a liquid containing extracts from several herbs, although juices, lotions, ointments, creams, powders, drops, tablets, capsules and suppositories may also be prescribed.

A BRIEF HISTORY

Currently enjoying a revival in popularity, herbal medicine's origins are lost in antiquity. There is now evidence as to the remarkable similarity of plant remedies used by different far-flung ancient civilisations. This would seem to indicate that the system originated as a result of a primitive instinct to seek out, or dowse, appropriate remedies for specific ailments. The first doctors—medicine men or 'wise women'—continue to look after some tribal cultures to this day.

Herbal medicine was used by several civilisations long before the birth of Christ; the earliest records are Chinese, dating back to 2800 BC. Hippocrates, known as the Father of Medicine, formulated the principle that treatment and dosage should be decided in accordance with the individual patient's requirements. This philosophy still holds true today.

The early Greeks were already using herbs from as far east as India, while the Roman conquest helped spread medical and herbal knowledge throughout Europe. Many new herbs arrived in Britain after the Roman invasion, and others as a result of trade with Mediterranean countries.

The advent of Christianity in the British Isles brought monks who used herbs from their physic gardens to treat themselves, the sick and the poor. Monasteries also doubled as medical training centres and hospitals. Also caring for the sick were ladies of the manor, who, in addition to preparing herbs for general use in the home, had the heavy responsibility of administering remedies to their family, household staff and the poor of the vicinity. This approach to healthcare did not alter significantly for several hundred years.

The work of the physician and alchemist Paracelsus (1493-1541) produced change and reform which had a far-reaching effect on healthcare. A firm believer in a return to the simplicity of the herbal system, Paracelsus also advocated the basic philosophy of homoeopathy, of treating like with like.

Impressive herbals were produced at the end of the sixteenth century by Gerade and fifty years later by the famous Nicholas Culpeper. At this time, different plants were arriving in Britain from the New World as a result of the settlers' continued herbal practice and their adoption of native plants used by the indigenous population.

Dr A. Coffin's reforms and dedicated efforts in the early part of the Victorian Age gave herbal medicine another boost and made it financially accessible to the majority of the population. However, in the latter half of the nineteenth century, increasing use was being made of the scientific process of isolating active properties from plants and later producing these ingredients synthetically. This practice formed the basis of modern conventional medicine and, with its rise, the simple herbal methods suffered a slide in popularity.

Today, almost one hundred years later, the demand for holistic healing methods has once again emphasised the efficacy of herbal medicine. Commercialisation and marketing have now taken herbal products into the public domain of the High Street.

The Herbal Practice

Members of the Institute of Medical Herbalists receive an extensive four-year training, which includes the study of anatomy and physiology. They also carry out simple medical diagnostic checks on patients.

An initial consultation can be expected to take about an hour. Respecting the individuality of each patient, the herbal practitioner will take a detailed, confidential case history in an endeavour to establish the cause of illness and any underlying imbalance. To help with the diagnosis, a routine examination may be necessary. In keeping with the 'whole person' philosophy, diet, nutrition and lifestyle will be discussed and rest and relaxation encouraged. Prescriptions are usually made up in the herbalist's dispensary. The length of a course of treatment will vary according to each patient's individual needs.

Preparation and Use of the Remedies

Most prescriptions given by herbalists are in the form of concentrated tinctures obtained by steeping fresh or dried herbs in a mixture of water and alcohol. They keep well. Syrups, creams and lotions have a tincture base. Infusions and decoctions, made on a daily basis, can easily be prepared at home as a self-help measure or under a practitioner's direction. An infusion, using the softer parts of plants, is made in much the same way as tea, using a teaspoon of fresh or 1/2 teaspoon of dried herbs to a cup of boiling water.

Decoction is the method required when the plants are of a more woody nature, or when nuts or seeds are being used. The herbs are placed in a saucepan, brought to the boil and simmered for ten to fifteen minutes before being used.

Dried herbs can be purchased from health food stores,

but fresh herbs may be dried easily at home. Picked in dry weather, at their best point of growth, in an area away from chemical pollutants and traffic fumes, the plants should be dried quickly in a warm, clean, airy place out of direct sunlight. When dry, the herbs should be stored in labelled, airtight containers.

HERBAL MEDICINE AND THE MENOPAUSE

Herbal medicine is extremely useful in treating menopausal symptoms. Probably the most distressing symptoms are those of hot flushes and night sweats. Their severity and frequency vary enormously between individuals. Stress is often an aggravating factor and therefore herbal treatment is aimed primarily at the nervous system. Herbs which are most useful include those listed below.

VALERIAN ROOT (VALERIANA OFFICINALIS)

This wild plant is found on dry heaths and high pastures and should not be confused with the red garden Valerian, which has no medicinal value. Valerian Root is well-known for its calming, tranquillising properties and is used in the treatment of anxiety, headaches, hot flushes, night sweats, insomnia and nervous tension. It is also of value where tension is held in the muscles, giving rise to symptoms such as cramp, digestive disorders and menstrual pain. Valerian Root will also reduce high blood pressure.

Self-treatment
Soak overnight before making a decoction. Take three times daily. Available in tablet or capsule form as directed.

MOTHERWORT (LEONURUS CARDIACA)

The fresh or dried aerial parts of this wild flower have been used for centuries in the treatment of problems relating to the female reproductive system, as a relaxant and heart tonic.

Symptoms assisted include hot flushes, night sweats and palpitations with anxiety and tension.

Self-treatment

An infusion taken three times daily. Available in tablet or capsule form as directed.

RED SAGE (SALVIA OFFICINALIS)

Also known as Purple Sage, this garden herb has a traditional link with longevity and has many medicinal uses. Its antiseptic properties prove effective in the treatment of sore throats and mouth infections when used in the form of a gargle. Red Sage is also beneficial in the treatment of digestive problems, nervous headaches and tension. One of several herbs containing oestrogen promoters, it is used to relieve menopausal hot flushes and night sweats.

Self-treatment

An infusion taken three times daily.

CHASTEBERRY (VITEX AGNUS-CASTUS)

Popularly known as Agnus Castus, this herb is of supreme importance in the treatment of menopausal problems and is an alternative to drugs for hormone imbalance. It does not contain oestrogen or progesterone, but acts on the pituitary gland, producing a regulatory, normalising effect. As hormone levels are at their most receptive in the morning (every woman ovulates in the morning), Agnus Castus is taken on rising.

The volatile oil of this herb acts on the anterior pituitary gland, reducing FSH (follicle stimulating hormone) and increasing the production of LSH (luteal stimulating hormone). It shifts the balance of oestrogen/progesterone towards a corpus luteum hormone effect. Excess FSH, which gives rise to pre-menstrual tension, is corrected by the use of Agnus Castus, as is LSH deficiency, which causes excessive bleeding. Agnus Castus acts as a precursor—it combines with other substances within the body to produce hormones.

Symptoms assisted include absence of periods, persistent bleeding between periods, heavy periods, pre-menstrual tension, painful breasts, recurrent mastitis. Available in tablet or capsule form as directed.

LIVER TONICS

The liver has an important role in monitoring hormonal health and is the principal organ responsible for eliminating unwanted substances from the body. The modern way of life puts pressure on the liver, requiring it to deal with numerous undesirable influences, including the effects of chemicals in food, environmental pollution, drugs and fat. Congestion is the result of the liver's failure to cope. Impaired liver function can manifest in symptoms such as:

• digestive disorders
• constipation/diarrhoea
• menstrual problems
• emotional debility
• sore eyes.

Herbs can play a valuable part in stimulating, strengthening and regenerating liver cells. Effective liver tonics include the following.

BURDOCK ROOT (ARCTIUM LAPPA)

This purifies the blood, helping to cleanse the body of accumulated toxins which can give rise to digestive disorders, skin problems and arthritic pain.

Dandelion Root (TARAXACUM OFFICINALE)

This is a cleansing, restorative tonic rich in minerals. A stimulant, it is a diuretic, mildly laxative and encourages bile flow. It assists calcium absorption, digestive function and many other conditions.

MILK THISTLE (CARDUUS MARIANUS)

This is a cleansing tonic and stimulant which helps to regenerate damaged liver cells. It protects against the effects of chemical stress, e.g. HRT and chemotherapy (during treatment).

ADRENAL AND BLOOD TONICS

Menstruating women tend to be blood deficient and can benefit from the help given by those herbs which encourage richness of blood.

During and after the menopause, as the production of oestrogen by the ovaries falls into a natural decline, the emphasis of responsibility for continued manufacture of oestrogen shifts primarily to the adrenal glands. Good adrenal health is therefore necessary to maintain an ongoing, adequate, balanced hormonal function. Effective adrenal and blood tonics include those outlined below.

LIQUORICE ROOT (GLYCYRRHIZA GLABRA)

This herb stimulates the adrenal glands, encouraging balanced hormonal production and anti-inflammatory action.

It relieves rheumatic pain, is helpful for chest infections and stomach ulcers and is mildly laxative.

Note Avoid where there is a history of high blood pressure. It might cause bloating and fluid retention.

Stinging Nettle (*Urtica dioica*)

This strengthens the adrenals and kidneys: the fresh plant restores and purifies the blood, helping acidic and toxic conditions. It cleanses and stimulates the circulation. Looked upon as a herbal tonic, as it is rich in vitamins, iron and many other minerals. Stinging nettle has a beneficial effect on the bones, skin, hair and nails. It has astringent (tightening) properties and reduces heavy menstrual bleeding.

Note The young leaves can be cooked like spinach.

Yellow Dock (*Rumex crispus*)

Yellow Dock cleanses the blood—its action encourages the absorption of iron and other minerals. It stimulates the flow of bile, is a diuretic and laxative.

Natural Hormone Precursors

These are listed below.

Black Cohosh (*Cimicifuga rucemosa*)
False Unicorn Root (*Chamoelirium luteum*)
Fennel (*Foeniculum vulgare*)
Ginseng (*Panax ginseng*)
Liquorice Root (*Glycyrrhiza glabra*)
Parsley (*Aphanes arvensis*)
Red Sage (*Salvia officinalis*)
Rosemary (*Rosemarinus officinalis*)

Sarsaparilla Root (*Smilax officinalis*)
Wild Yam (*Dioscorea villasa*)

NERVINE HERBS
These are for conditions such as fatigue, depression, insomnia and cramp.

Chamomile (*Matricaria recutita*) Sedative, relaxing, for tension causing digestive problems.
Hops (*Humulus lupulus*) Soothes digestive and nervous system, sedative.
Lemon Balm (*Melissa officinalis*) Anti-depressant, for nervous tension, relaxes digestive and nervous system.
Note Promotes perspiration.
Lime Blossom (*Tilia cordata*) Relaxing.
Passionflower (*Passiflora incarnata*) Sedative, relaxing, for muscle tension.
Rosemary (*Rosemarinus officinalis*) For fatigue, relaxing, tonic, also acts on circulation.
Valerian Root (*Valeriana officinalis*) Relaxing, for nervous tension, muscle cramp, sedative.

HERBS WHICH BENEFIT THE FEMALE REPRODUCTIVE SYSTEM AND HELP REDUCE SYMPTOMS
Angelica Root (*Angelica archangelica*) Warming digestive and blood tonic, for anaemia, menstrual irregularities and painful periods (dysmenorrhoea).
False Unicorn Root (*Chamoelirium luteum*) Hormonal regulator, useful following hysterectomy, tonic, heavy periods.
Ladies Mantle (*Alchemilla vulgaris*) Regulates excessive

bleeding, painful periods.

Parsley (*Aphanes arvensis*) Rich in iron—helpful in anaemia—strengthens digestive system.

Raspberry Leaf (*Rubus ideaus*) Tones uterus and eases menstrual discomfort.

Yarrow (*Achilla millefolium*) For heavy periods, incontinence, improves circulation.

Note Can promote perspiration with hot flushes.

CASE HISTORIES

MARILYN

Believing at fifty-two that she was too old to be troubled by menopausal symptoms, Marilyn was distressed when she started experiencing incessant hot flushes and night sweats. Married, with two grown-up sons, she was working full-time as secretary to the managing director of a large company. Marilyn was normally a happy person with no real worries. However, she found that lack of sleep and daytime discomfort and embarrassment were affecting her work performance. She felt tense, upset and tired.

Marilyn saw a medical herbalist whose routine examination established that her general health was good, but that she had a tendency to constipation. Dietary changes were recommended : Marilyn's diet was lacking in fresh fruit, salads and vegetables. She was eating too much protein, particularly meat and meat products. A wholefood diet was advised, reducing meat and increasing roughage.

Herbalist Prescribed

Vitex Agnus Castus fluid extract. Ten drops on rising.

Valerian Root (*Valeriana officinalis*) As a relaxant.

Motherwort (*Leonurus cardiaca*) and **Red Sage** (*Salvia officinalis*) Both specifically for hot flushes.
Dandelion Root (*Taraxacum radix*) Liver tonic.

After five weeks, Marilyn's symptoms disappeared and there has been no recurrence.

ELIZABETH

Elizabeth had worked as a hairdresser since leaving school and had recently invested most of her savings in opening her own salon in partnership with a colleague. Despite much hard work put in by both of them, the business had been slow to establish itself and Elizabeth was feeling worried that she may have been unwise to embark on the venture.

There were also problems at home. Elizabeth's husband was unhappy in his work and had become very difficult to live with. In addition, one of their two teenage children had been stealing at school.

Recalling that one of her customers had been very enthusiastic about the help she had received at the time of the menopause from a medical herbalist, Elizabeth went for a consultation. She was then aged forty-seven.

The presenting symptoms formed quite a list:
* menstruation—the cycle was becoming shorter, lasting twenty to twenty-two days
* irritable bowel syndrome—history of constipation, now experiencing alternating constipation and diarrhoea
* stress
* recurrent sinus problems
* back pain—recent X-rays revealed some osteoporosis.

On questioning Elizabeth about her diet, the herbalist found she was eating mainly convenience foods. She needed to reduce fat, protein— particularly meat—sugar and coffee. The function of the parathyroid gland, which regulates calcium metabolism, would benefit from raw fruit and vegetables.

The benefits of regular exercise, such as brisk walking, swimming, stationary bicycling and aerobic dancing were stressed. As Elizabeth had never taken much exercise, she decided to make time for a daily walk in the country.

Herbs Prescribed
Yarrow (*Achillea millefolium*) To lengthen the menstrual cycle.
Chamomile (*Matricaria*) For the irritable bowel syndrome.
Valerian Root (*Valeriana officinalis*) For the stress.
Elderflower (*Sambucus*) For the sinuses.

Elizabeth's menstrual cycle immediately regulated. Now fifty-one, her periods are still occurring every twenty-seven to twenty-eight days. The problems with her bowels cleared and there is now no tendency to constipation. She has not suffered any more sinus problems. The benefits of the healthy diet and regular exercise also became apparent, and Elizabeth began to feel fitter and more able to cope with the pressures of business and home. The whole family were helped by the dietary changes.

JEAN

Jean had last seen her medical herbalist when she was forty. She had been in good health until she was forty-nine, when her menstrual cycle changed. Twelve months later, on consulting the herbalist again, she complained that her periods had become very heavy and irregular. There was no pain, but some PMT, particularly irritability.

Jean worked as a dental receptionist and was worried about her short-tempered attitude with the patients. Normally calm and easy-going, she was often irritable at home with her husband and three children.

Although her diet was reasonably good—wholefood with some meat, high in fruit, low in fat, salt and sugar—she was advised by the herbalist to make some adjustments and especially to increase green and other vegetables. More exercise was recommended.

Apart from her irritability, Jean reported that emotionally she felt quite balanced and happy. Jean also complained of varicose veins in both legs with some oedema around both ankles. This was bothering her at work where she was on her feet quite a lot.

Herbs Prescribed

Vitex Agnus Castus fluid extract Ten drops on rising (Vitex Agnus Castus is a hormone regulator, affecting the pituitary gland, and is particularly useful for pre-menstrual symptoms).

For the menorrhagia (heavy bleeding):
Lady's Mantle (*Alchemilla vulgaris*)
Beth Root (*Trillium erectum*)
Pasque Flower (*Anemone pulsatilla*) Sedative to uterus.

For the varicose veins:
Horsechestnut (*Aesculus hippocastaneum*)
Dandelion Leaf (*Taraxacum herba*)
Prickly Ash Bark (*Zanthoxylum*)

After one month's treatment, Jean's periods became much lighter. After two months, the pre-menstrual symptoms disappeared. The varicose veins are feeling more comfortable, although there has been no visible change.

CHAPTER ELEVEN

Homoeopathy

WHAT IS HOMOEOPATHY?

Homoeopathy (pronounced hom-ee-opathy) is a system of natural medicine which is based upon the principle of similars: let like treat like. It is also a system of healing which treats the whole person, and is as concerned with the maintenance of good health as with treating bad health. In addition, homoeopathy relies upon the body's own ability to heal itself. The role of homoeopathy is to cure the sick, not the disease itself.

The present-day success of homoeopathy can be attributed to several factors:

- it is effective as a first-aid measure and in treating both acute and more deep-seated illness
- its action is gentle and safe, the remedies inexpensive to administer
- the absence of side-effects and toxicity make it a desirable option in the treatment of children, adults and animals
- increasing numbers of dentists and veterinary surgeons are now also using the system.

A BRIEF HISTORY

The word homoeopathy is derived from the Greek words *homoios* and *pathos*, meaning 'similar suffering'. Its practice has been riding high on the wave of public interest over the last fifteen years or so, but it is not a new therapy. The homoeopathic approach has links with the ancient Ayurvedic healing system of India. Hippocrates treated patients in the fifth century using the similars principle, as did Paracelsus in the fifteenth and sixteenth centuries, but it was not until the middle of the eighteenth century that Samuel Hahnemann took up the theory again, researched it and put it into practice.

Samuel Hahnemann (1755–1843) was a doctor practising in Germany, who had become disillusioned with medical practices at that time. These consisted mainly of purging and routine bleeding of patients, using leeches. He felt that there must be a better way of restoring patients to health and began a series of experiments on himself, his family and a loyal band of helpers.

Hahnemann observed that when he took quinine in large doses, he developed all the signs and symptoms of marsh fever (malaria). When the medicine was stopped, all these signs and symptoms disappeared, only to reappear if the medicine was taken again. As quinine was used to treat marsh fever, he was obviously fascinated by this phenomenon. He then went on to take himself, and give to others, large doses of other substances in use at the time, observing and documenting all the signs and symptoms which were produced.

Samuel Hahnemann used many people in his 'provings' of remedies. None experienced lasting ill effects; in fact, he established that the prover's health was improved as a result. He then went on to use this information to treat patients, with great success, using the principle of similars: if a substance would produce a symptom, it would also cure that symptom.

However, in the course of treating people, he noticed that

although they did fully recover, they got worse before they got better. In order to reduce this 'aggravation', Hahnemann began to dilute the remedies and, in doing so, found that he was able to effect a cure without producing an initial aggravation. The process he used is called potentisation.

HOMOEOPATHY TODAY

The reaction of the medical establishment of the day to Samuel Hahnemann's research work and practical application of the method was unsupportive and obstructive. However, the popularity of homoeopathy grew, spreading throughout Europe, to America and Great Britain. With the arrival of modern medicine, homoeopathy, together with herbalism, took a place in the wings until the recent revival of interest. Today, the spread of homoeopathy has continued and it is now practised in many countries worldwide. The British royal family has a long tradition of using homoeopathic treatment.

In Britain, there is a small but rapidly increasing number of doctors who have studied homoeopathy and are using it either privately or through the NHS. Some doctors may have had only a short training and have little practical experience. Ask about their background if you are unsure. There is also a body of practitioners who undergo very extensive training in homoeopathy and who practise as professional homoeopaths. Although not medically qualified, they will, if appropriate, work in close cooperation with GPs.

Homoeopathy does not disregard the notable advances made by medical science, or claim to be a panacea. But it has stood the test of time, proving that homoeopath and patient can work together to achieve lasting benefits for the patient.

HOMOEOPATHIC REMEDIES

There are over 2000 remedies from which the homoeopath can choose. Though derived from many sources, most of the remedies come from plants and minerals. Full details of remedies are found in reference books called homoeopathic *materia medica*. The process of 'proving' new remedies is continuing.

Remedies are prepared by a process of dilution and succussion—a process of vigorous shaking described by Hahnemann. A tincture of the remedy is prepared by immersion in alcohol. One drop of the filtered liquid is then added to ninety-nine drops of water and shaken. Then one drop of this solution is taken and added to ninety-nine drops of water and the mixture is shaken again. The process is continued until the desired dilution is reached; the dilutions commonly used are the sixth and thirtieth. The remedy will therefore be labelled 6c or 30c; the higher the figure, the more potent the remedy.

BUYING REMEDIES

The lower potencies (6c and 30c) can be bought over the counter from health food shops and most chemists. Higher potencies (best administered by a practitioner) and tinctures for external use are available from homoeopathic pharmacies. Many pharmacies also have a mail order service. Most remedies are taken in tablet or pillule form, though some are sometimes prescribed as powders or granules.

TAKING REMEDIES

The remedies are sensitive to smells and strong flavours, particularly peppermint and coffee, which can have a detrimental effect on their action. It is therefore advisable to avoid handling them, or allowing them to come into contact with flavours in the mouth. The remedies, which have a pleasant taste, should be taken from the lid of the container and tipped straight onto the tongue where they should be allowed to dissolve. The palate should be clean—avoid eating, drinking or cleaning the teeth half an hour either side of taking a remedy.

ENERGY MEDICINE

Although many substances used to make homoeopathic remedies are poisonous in their natural state, e.g. deadly nightshade (Belladonna), arsenic (Arsenicum) and snake venom (Lachesis), the process of dilution past a certain very low potency means none of the original substance remains in the resulting remedy.

THE HOMOEOPATHIC CONSULTATION

Homoeopathy can be placed high in the list of holistic therapies and the consultation reflects this. An initial consultation routinely takes between one and one and a half hours. Its purpose is to determine the patient's present complaints and what might have contributed to them.

The homoeopath will be interested in your past and family medical history, the timing of illnesses in relation to life events, social circumstances and how you function and relate to the world and other people. You will be asked questions about your likes and dislikes, emotional temperament, fears, anxieties, when or what makes the symptoms better or worse, reaction to weather changes and many other things.

The homoeopath will endeavour to relate all this information to the wealth of clinical material gathered in the provings of remedies to try to find one remedy which fits your symptom picture—the general, emotional and specific physical symptoms of which you are complaining. The chosen medication is usually given in a single dose and is sometimes known as the constitutional remedy. This method of prescribing is recognised as being the most effective method of treatment. The constitutional remedy has the ability to treat on all levels, and so achieves a better re-balancing of the body energies.

Much of the responsibility for the healing process lies with you, the patient, and you should be open to advice which may be offered by the practitioner on diet, lifestyle, etc. You will be expected to observe, note and report changes in symptoms or the development of new symptoms to the homoeopath at your next meeting. Your case will be re-assessed, with perhaps the same remedy being given again, or a new remedy prescribed.

SELF-TREATMENT

Homoeopathy can be successfully used in self-treatment for many common ailments or specific problems. However, the treatment of serious or more complicated problems is best left in the hands of a qualified practitioner. When using homoeopathy at home, a few simple rules should be observed:

- where applicable, match, as closely as possible, your symptoms and personality to the symptoms picture of the remedy
- do not take more than one remedy at a time
- take only the minimum dose and lowest potency required.

As homoeopathy works slowly and gently, instant results
should not be anticipated. Homoeopathy has its own
philosophy and laws like any other science. Recovery is
governed by Hering's Law of Cure which is used as a
yardstick by homoeopaths when monitoring their patients'
progress. In brief, this says:

(a) healing takes place from the inside to the outside
(b) it goes from vital to less vital organs
(c) it often follows a downward direction, from head to foot
(d) the first symptoms to appear will be the last to be cured
     (they may return briefly, then disappear again).

USING HOMOEOPATHY TO TREAT THE MENOPAUSE

The imbalances experienced at menopause are often
indications of problems which have been present for a long
time. Treating the whole symptom picture constitutionally
using a single remedy is the most effective path. Some
homeopathic remedies tend to be more suited to women
who suffer a multitude of symptoms in the peri-menopausal
period and are often prescribed for this. The most commonly
used remedies have long lists of signs and symptoms
attributed to them in the *materia medica*, but the relevant
symptoms for each remedy are summarised below.

SEPIA (*THE INK OF THE CUTTLEFISH*)

This is a commonly used remedy, which is especially helpful
to women. It has been called 'the homeopathic hormone re-
balancer'.

Key Symptoms

Poor memory, difficulty in concentrating

Weepiness (including when recounting symptoms), changeable moods; better for a good cry

Indifference to loved ones

Irritability

Hair loss

Heavy periods with flooding

Irregular periods

Hot sweats; worse at night

General exhaustion and weariness

Low backache; better for pressure and exercise

Bearing down sensation, must sit down and cross legs

Flushes and sweats, especially on back, armpits and genitals

Chilliness

Averse to sympathy, but dreads being alone

Faints easily

Desires vinegar and spices, averse to meat and milk.

SULPHUR

One of the great homoeopathic remedies, used extensively since Hahnemann's day.

Key Symptoms

Poor memory

Depression

Indifference to others

Indifferent to own appearance

Craving for sweet things, especially pre-menstrually

Hot sweats day and night

Dry itchy skin

Generally hot

Flushes; worse in the evenings

Redness

Burning sensations

Tendency to put on weight.

LACHESIS (*VENOM OF THE BUSHMASTER SNAKE*)
Key Symptoms
Poor memory
Difficulty in concentrating
Hot flushes around the head, neck and face
Heavy, irregular periods
Sleeplessness; wakes feeling worse
All symptoms worse for the failure of an expected discharge,
i.e. when periods finally stop or pre-menstrually
Symptoms relate to the left side of the body
All symptoms worse for heat
All symptoms worse in spring and mild rainy weather
Symptoms related to head and neck
Unable to tolerate tight clothing
Jealous, suspicious
Extremely talkative.

PULSATILLA (*THE WIND FLOWER*)
Key Symptoms
Depression and weepiness
Mood swings
Pre-menstrual headache
Perspiration and observable sweating on face
Tendency to vaginal infection and discharge
Hot offensive sweats; worse at night
Mild, yielding disposition
Suspicious, jealous, peevish and irritable
Likes to be shown sympathy
Aversion to the opposite sex, but likes to be cuddled
Worse in a warm, stuffy room, but can be chilly in a warm
room
Worse in the evenings

Much better for being in the open air
Absence of thirst
Desires sweet foods, but rich food disagrees.

CALCEREA (MIDDLE LAYER OF THE OYSTER SHELL)
Key Symptoms
Poor memory
Irritability, depression, weepiness
Headache, worse before a period
Perspiration on head and sometimes on face
Swelling of finger joints
Legs go to sleep
Cramps and twitching in calves
Vaginal discharge
Very chilly
Fat and flabby
Worse for cold, especially damp cold
Sluggish
Anxious about future health
Desires eggs.

GRAPHITES (BLACK LEAD)
Key Symptoms
Irresolute
Indecisive
Poor concentration
Heavy, irregular periods
Dryness of the vagina
Offensive sweats
Tendency to flush
Timid and apprehensive
Weeps, especially on hearing music

Difficulty in getting to sleep at night due to mental activity
Chilly, pale, fat and flabby
Averse to sweets and fish.

PHOSPHORUS
Key Symptoms
Poor memory
Over-excitable
Mood swings, either very high or very low
Sleeplessness
Profuse sweats on exertion or in bed in the mornings
Sweat on upper lip on exertion or mental exercise
Heavy, bright red menses
Fatigued and weary
Full of fear, especially of thunder, the dark, death
Indifferent to loved ones
Craves sympathy and loves to be touched
Artistic and intuitive
Chilly—loves the sunshine
Desires ice cold drinks and salt
Head and stomach symptoms are better for cold, all other symptoms are better for warmth
All symptoms improved by sleep, even a catnap.

These remedies are used to treat the specific menopausal symptoms as noted, but if the remedy is well chosen on the whole symptom picture, it will also treat other problems which occur around the menopause but may not be strictly due to ovarian failure. It is usually worth the time and effort to decide upon the best remedy match.

Homoeopathy can also be used to help those who have suffered adverse reaction to HRT, but treatment in such cases is best handled by a practitioner.

CASE HISTORIES

ANGELA

Angela gave the homoeopath doctor a long list of complaints at their initial consultation and told her that she felt sure all her problems were due to stress. She was aged forty-seven, married to a teacher and they had two teenage children. She was employed as a social worker and six months previously, due to her husband's job being threatened, had started working full-time. Her daughter had just had a nervous breakdown and her father-in-law had recently died.

There was nothing of note in Angela's medical history until she was in her early forties. At forty-three, she had had a hysterectomy, with conservation of both ovaries. This was because she had been experiencing heavy and continuous bleeding due to the presence of uterine fibroids. She had received no subsequent treatment. There was nothing of particular note in Angela's family medical history.

Angela's Complaints

The homoeopath listed Angela's complaints as follows. She had been feeling ill for four months and felt she had only half her usual energy, physically and mentally. She felt permanently tired and wanted to sit down all the time. She ached all over. Six weeks previous to the consultation, she had an acute episode of severe indigestion, accompanied by severe pain in the rectum. This was constant and unremitting and she felt that something was lodged in her gullet. She was better for eating small amounts of food, but the pain returned after five to six minutes. Despite this, she had no change in bowel habits. She felt that her memory and concentration were deteriorating. Her skin had become dry and itchy. She had noticed that she was bruising easily. She was feeling the cold more than ever; there were no flushes or sweats. She had developed low backache for the first time since pregnancy.

The homoeopath was guided by the following homoeopathic pointers. Angela was weepy, especially when relating her symptoms. She suddenly, for the first time in her life, could not tolerate being left alone. Her relationship with her husband was suffering, as she was so tired and irritable; in addition, she was not able to contemplate any sexual relationship. She felt angry, frustrated and resentful.

All her symptoms were worse on waking and she was increasingly feeling that she could not face the day. All symptoms were worse for being cold. She was unable to discuss how she felt with anyone, as she was frightened that she would begin to weep. Her taste for foods had changed. She had lost her desire for dairy products and now wanted tasty, spicy food.

TREATMENT

Sepia 30c was given for ten days, with marked improvement in her emotional state and energy levels. The indigestion disappeared. The improvement continued, and after a period of six weeks, Angela was able to accept counselling to help with the obvious psychological causative factors, which were also affecting her physical health. She is now content, and feeling well and takes a maintenance dose of Sepia each month.

PATRICIA

Patricia consulted a homoeopathic doctor at the age of fifty, feeling particularly worried about hot flushes and sweats which had become unbearably severe. She was a busy career woman, managing a small business. Her husband ran his own business. They had been married for twenty-five years and there were no children. There was nothing significant to note in Patricia's past medical history or in that of her family.

Patricia had started her periods at fifteen years of age, and the cycle had always been regular. (She had taken the Pill for fifteen years, but had been off it in later years.) Her periods had always been painful, but not too heavy. She had had no pregnancies. Three years before, her periods had become scantier, and eighteen months previously she had started to miss the odd bleed. She had not had a period for six months.

Patricia's Complaints

The homoeopath listed Patricia's complaints as follows.

Six months previously, she had started to have hot flushes and sweats. They had been present for some years, but had become unbearable in the past six months. The flushes normally started in the face and spread to the neck area, with redness and sweating. They happened at any time but tended to be worse in bed, and would wake her. She had begun to feel irritable and insecure in her marriage and in her job because she felt that she might be replaced by a younger woman. This feeling was reinforced by the fact that she knew that her concentration and memory were not as good as before and she felt that she was less efficient.

She had generalised aches and pains, but particularly painful swollen small joints in the left hand. She had started to take too much alcohol as it made her feel better. She did not like being too hot, as she felt this could trigger a hot flush. She no longer wanted to sunbathe, as this produced a headache. (This was a source of anxiety as she and her husband had previously gone for their holidays to exotic places.)

The homoeopath was guided by the following homoeopathic pointers.

Patricia was very articulate and did not withhold any information. In fact, she found talking about her problems very easy. She now hated both very hot and very cold weather and dreaded springtime because she felt things were worse then. She wanted to wear fewer clothes, and had given away her high-necked jumpers.

She felt that she was tempted to eat more and that she was putting on weight. She found dieting particularly difficult and was craving sweets and chocolate. She was obviously sleeping less well, was tired all the time and was having difficulty with concentration and memory. These symptoms had got much worse since her periods had stopped.

Treatment

Lachesis 30c, 200c, 1m (ascending dose per day for three days). This gave a great improvement and made the flushes bearable. She also felt better emotionally and generally. The improvement was maintained for four months and then the symptoms began to creep back. A follow-up dose of Lachesis 1m x 3 has kept Patricia well until the present day.

CHAPTER TWELVE

Meditation

WHAT IS MEDITATION?

Meditation is a state of relaxed, wakeful awareness which enables the mind to rest and be still in a way that transcends the everyday world. Many different disciplines and techniques can be employed to bring this about, from concentrating on an object, your breath, a word or a sound.

In this altered state of consciousness, feelings of inner knowing, clarity and peace are promoted. The heart and mind can tune in, not only to itself, but to the larger picture of life. Meditation helps to develop a deeper way of thinking and feeling; to explore the power of the self beyond the conscious personality; to tap into the resources of wisdom and truth within that help us to grow. Negative patterns of thought and behaviour are left behind, as more positive qualities and viewpoints emerge. The body is allowed to heal itself in whatever way is needed. Changing values and increased freedom invite the exploration of fresh opportunities. The achievement of more satisfying goals can be realised.

Regular, sincere meditation can bring many benefits to the body and mind. It is of particular value in stress-related and emotional problems. It provides an opportunity to move on, to develop or gain qualities such as confidence, contentment, acceptance, tranquillity and the most elusive quality of all—inner happiness. Many activities, given the right circumstances, awareness and attitude, could be classed as meditations in themselves. You can be quite unaware that you are meditating when enjoying everyday activities like listening to music, gardening, sewing or dancing.

The more formal practices, often associated with mysticism and the path to enlightenment, have been followed since early times. They were used by ancient civilisations, religions and esoteric groups as part of rituals and healing practices. Indeed, most religions today have a form of meditation or contemplation embedded in their spiritual foundations. The Oriental practice of Transcendental Meditation became fashionable in the West in the 1960s, and is now widely recognised for its therapeutic value as a truly holistic practice (embracing the concept that the body, mind and spirit are inseparable). The practice of meditation is not confined to those following particular forms of religion, mysticism or philosophy and can be done without difficulty by anyone.

WHAT HAPPENS DURING MEDITATION?

The body's response whilst meditating is different from that during sleep or hypnosis. In physiological terms, in meditation the metabolic rate is lowered. The heart rate slows and there is a decrease in blood pressure. Blood lactate levels (connected with anxiety) drop. Breathing becomes more regular and subtle, as a result of a reduced oxygen requirement. The brain produces alpha waves, a wave frequency associated with deep relaxation, tranquillity of the mind and emotions, day-dreaming and self-healing.

Within the alpha wave band, there are smaller bands which work to heal and balance various functions of the body such as pain control and the hormonal system. A relaxed state produces more alpha waves than a tense one.

The more alpha waves transmitted, the better you will feel.

Changes which occur during meditation also affect the hypothalamus in the brain. This important gland, which is particularly sensitive during the time of menopause, is concerned with keeping the body in balance. It acts as the master controller—regulating, mediating and overseeing functions such as the menstrual cycle, water balance, body temperature, emotional health and desires, appetite, sleep patterns, the autonomic nervous system and reactions to stress. Given the stimulus of meditation, the hypothalamus comes into play, directing the body's reaction, adjustment and finer balance.

Meditation nourishes and rejuvenates every cell in the body, encouraging and extending its growth and slowing down the ageing process. During meditation, the body enters a timeless state and is unaware of conscious reality. It feels expanded, yet centred. Sensations of tingling or slight numbness are sometimes felt. Colours or visions may be seen, or the voice of intuition heard. Upon completing a meditation, there is a feeling of being grounded. The mind feels revitalised, yet still.

MEDITATION AND THE MENOPAUSE

Women suffering from stress-related ailments can benefit from meditation. Many symptoms attributed to the menopause and pre-menstrual syndrome can be helped. Although there have been some changes in our national attitude, Britain, on the whole, remains true to its stiff upper lip image. Difficulty in coping with stress is still to a large extent considered a stigma and hidden from others. The atmosphere in the workplace tends to be increasingly insecure, cut-throat and uncaring. Most women need to work, but fear that admitting to being depressed or having other emotional problems will appear as a blot on their employment record, perhaps ruining chances of promotion or leading to redundancy.

The capacity to listen to the inner voice, understand and share problems with others can develop through meditation. The symptoms or signals offered at the time of menopause are cries for help, attention and change. In heeding the signals, doors open, providing opportunities for true creativity and wisdom to flow. The accomplishment of an inspired way of living is only a step away.

PHYSICAL BENEFITS

The physical benefits of meditation are that it:

- reduces time needed for sleep. Just half an hour's meditation can lessen sleep requirement by up to two hours
- assists restful sleep and prevents insomnia
- rejuvenates. Slows cell activity and protects against senility
- lowers blood pressure
- brings relief in many stress-related ailments, such as asthma, migraines and ulcers.

MENTAL BENEFITS

The mental benefits are that it:

- develops clarity of mind
- brings confidence
- relaxes, balances and re-energises
- promotes increased self-awareness, allowing the loving qualities of empathy, kindness and acceptance to be enjoyed

- makes problem-solving easier
- balances the emotions. Assists in the release of trapped feelings such as fear, anger and other blocks which prevent good health
- encourages positive thought, prevents depression
- improves communication and relationships with others
- heightens the senses
- keeps the brain active, enabling it to maintain concentration and focus
- brings inner peace and joy
- develops the intuition and creativity.

Menopause provides an opportunity for a re-think and spring-clean on an inner level. Working at your own pace, meditation and visualisation provide a gentle method of facing up to and understanding personal distress. You will, most likely, emerge feeling you are a much nicer person to know.

Regular meditation practice can bring about a state of forgiveness. It can create an environment for the inner release of unwanted ties, patterns, old hurts, fears, anxieties and resentments. A release, or catharsis, will take place at the time and in the manner which is right for you. It may be by way of tears, a bodily sensation, a feeling of lightness or it may be so subtle as to go unnoticed.

There are numerous ways of utilising meditation in healing, including breathing techniques, symbolic visualisations and the use of colour. Sadly, the space in this section only provides room for a little help, but you can investigate further by reading, attending workshops and trying meditation for yourself.

PRACTISING MEDITATION

Meditation can be practised alone or in groups of any size. Initially it could be helpful to join a small group, where you are likely to find good advice and support. Group meditations are normally organised meetings, with a leader taking a guided programme. An advantage of working in a group is the availability of increased 'energy' for use by the whole group.

Meditating alone offers you the convenience of being at home or in a place of your personal choice, not being tied to a programme or routine and being able to practise in whatever way feels right at the time.

For meditation to be effective, it has to be practised on a regular basis, preferably every day, and if possible twice daily. Traditionally, meditation is done at dawn and dusk. If meditating twice a day, leave at least six hours between practices. If possible, keep to a regular time of day and start with fifteen to twenty minutes a time.

Choose a place which is restful to you, ensuring as far as possible that you will not be disturbed, and reserve it for your practice. By using the same space each time, you will find yourself more readily able to enter a meditative state. In warmer weather it is pleasant to meditate in a garden or peaceful place outdoors. You may prefer to play some restful music or burn a candle or oils while meditating, perhaps making a focal point of a small table or shelf, placing upon it items such as flowers, a picture which has special meaning, crystals or a symbol of your choice. Some people feel benefit from holding a crystal during their practice.

Remember that the body must remain still during practice, so it is important to feel comfortable and relaxed before starting; wear loose clothing and remove your shoes. It is important to remember that your back should be kept as straight as possible during meditation and that no part of your body should feel strained. The traditional Lotus position cannot be considered a beginner's posture, and it is not necessary to struggle to do it in order to meditate successfully. A few simple suggested sitting positions are illustrated. For the cross-legged and Burmese sitting positions, try sitting on one or two cushions. Hands can be cupped, kept loose and placed with palms up or down on the thighs or knees, or held palms up in the traditional Oriental chin mudra. In this position, the thumb and forefinger are lightly pressed together. It is said that this seals the energy circuit flowing through the body. It is a good idea to run through a short relaxation routine first, such as deep breathing.

When you are feeling settled, close your eyes and take some deep relaxing breaths. Breathe in, and on the out-breath, imagine a silver stream of energy flowing from the top of your head, through your body and out through the soles of your feet deep into the ground. Breathe normally to a steady rhythm. You are now in a position to start your chosen meditation technique or routine.

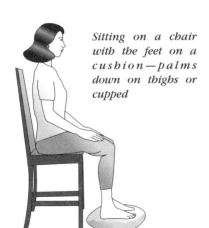

Sitting on a chair with the feet on a cushion—palms down on thighs or cupped

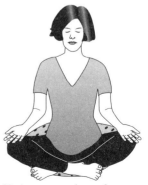

Sitting cross-legged on a cushion—palms up (loosley) resting on knees

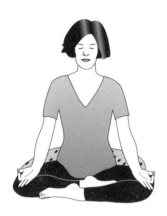

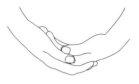

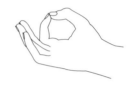

Close-up of hand positions: cupped, and chin mudra.

Sitting in the Burmese posture on a cushion—palms up on knees in chin mudra position

LOSING CONCENTRATION

The mind is not easy to control. It is quite natural for it to stray and for thoughts or feelings to disturb a meditation. If this happens, simply acknowledge the thought or feeling, let it go and return to your chosen method of concentration.

CREATIVE VISUALISATION AND THE USE OF COLOUR

Best done in a relaxed or meditative state, the practice of creative visualisation utilises the subconscious mind to accomplish positive improvements in health, attitudes, lifestyle and relationships. In creative visualisation, the conscious imagination is used as a tool for programming the subconscious mind, by creating images or symbols of things you wish to have or experience. It is not necessary to hold spiritual beliefs in order to use creative visualisation effectively, but it is important to be positive about what you wish to achieve.

Creative visualisation is very easy. Simply relax into a peaceful state, set yourself a desired goal or scene, which can be real or imagined, still or moving. Immerse yourself in the imagery and remain focused on it. Trust that the outcome, which might not always happen in exactly the way you envisage, will be to the highest good. The potential for positive change is enormous. Scenes and walks in nature, utilising its colours, symbols and energy, are particularly useful in physical and emotional healing. Take your time to explore your imagined environment; admiring the beauty, observing colours, smells, hearing sounds, feeling textures and the sun or breeze on your skin.

Hot flushes and overwrought conditions can be helped with imagery using cooling scenes and colours: snow-clad mountains, icebergs in a blue sea, winter sunshine in a clear blue sky.

The nervous and physical problems of the menopause can be ameliorated by using the relaxing, balancing colour of green. Sit or walk in a meadow or garden. A tree, when used in creative visualisation, has a strengthening and grounding effect on the body; take a walk along a woodland path, enjoy the glinting rays of the sun through the trees.

Scenes involving flowing water can be used when the mind is bothered by negative thoughts, bitterness and frustration; put your feet into the water and release the negativity. Try visualising sailing ships on water, which will help problems to be seen from a more positive perspective. If you are feeling very depleted, gently introduce a waterfall into your visualisation.

The Waterfall—A Self-Healing Visualisation
Begin by closing your eyes and relaxing into the breath.

Imagine you are enjoying a walk though a small meadow. You feel the warmth of the spring sunshine on your head. The long grass shimmers in the gentle breeze. You listen to the birds singing and watch butterflies dancing over the beautiful wild flowers.

You see a small Turkish-style carpet lying on the ground a little way ahead. Admire its colours and pattern, walk towards it and sit down to rest. The carpet slowly rises into the air and moves off over the meadow. You look down as the carpet gains height, passing over fields, forests, hills, towns and villages. You see rivers and streams winding their way through the countryside. Fluffy white clouds float by.

On being joined by swooping seagulls, you look around for the sea. A harbour, bustling with fishing boats, comes into view. You travel on over the deep blue water, seeing ships and boats, passing small islands. Ahead you see a long, empty, sandy beach; a range of tree-clad hills rises behind it. Passing over the hills, you sense the carpet descending and look down at an enchanting valley, at one end of which there is a tumbling, golden waterfall.

The carpet gently settles you onto the lush grass nearby. Moving towards the waterfall, you see that it is made of golden light energy. Step into it. Enjoy the feelings of warmth and security, of healing energy flowing through every atom of your body. Send that healing light to any part of you that needs it; know that the problem is melting away.

Say to yourself: 'I release all negative feelings and dissolve all disharmony.' Imagine you are now in perfect health. Remain in the waterfall a few moments longer, breathing the golden energy, then slowly walk away; return to your carpet, sit down, take one last look at the lovely waterfall. Pass over the hills to the sea again, on and on, enjoying a feeling of peace and contentment. See the harbour and countryside below. Feel the carpet slowly descending and watch as you come to rest in the same meadow where you began your journey. Give thanks and leave the carpet.

CLOSING DOWN

The process of grounding is an important part of meditation, as it maintains your link with the earth. There are many ways, including the use of sound, to connect with the earth. A suggested routine for grounding and gently closing down your meditation practice is as follows.

Be aware of your energy, of how expanded you feel and yet how centred and secure. On the next few out-breaths, imagine a silver stream of energy flowing from the top of your head, through your body, down your legs and out through your feet into the ground. Think of your favourite tree. See it with its leaves turning brown in autumn. Know that, as the roots go down, the branches reach out and the tree is in balance. Start to be aware of where you are sitting and the room around you. Starting to move gently, rub your hands together, rub your knees, have a good stretch, open your eyes and, when you are ready, get up slowly.

SIMPLE MEDITATION TECHNIQUE

A ten minute exercise for beginners. Try the very simple routine of breath counting.

- Feel that you are in a relaxed, peaceful state.
- After breathing for a while in a relaxed rhythm, breath in and on the out breath mentally count one.

Breath in and count two on the out breath. Carry on up to ten; then reverse the process, counting down from nine to one on each out breath.

- If you lose your way with the counting, return to one and carry on as before.
- When you are ready, close down the meditation in the manner suggested or in a way which is comfortable for you.

WATCHING THE BREATH

Probably the most powerful, yet simple, meditation of all is the Buddhist practice of watching the breath.

- Feel that you are in a relaxed, peaceful state.
- Breathing normally, in a relaxed manner, focus the mind on the area of the chest; feel its rise and fall with each breath.
- After a few minutes bring the attention to the nose. Feel the breath going in and out of the nostrils and the sensation as it reaches the skin of the upper lip area.
- Remain focused on the nose area and continue to observe the breath entering and leaving the nostrils for a few more minutes.
- When you are ready, close down the meditation in a way which is comfortable to you.

If the mind wanders during this practice, breathing more heavily will assist the mind to return to the concentration.

AFFIRMATIONS

Affirmations are clear, positive statements of intent, used

independently at any time, during meditation or in support of methods of creative visualisation. They can be written, thought or spoken aloud. Affirmations are not intended to alter your character and emotional make-up. Instead, their aim is to encourage you to develop a more positive attitude to life. You can choose to use the process to create better health, extend limited horizons and attract a more rewarding way of living.

Affirmations are made in the present tense—using the word 'now' in your statement is helpful. The end result will come more easily if you keep your statements brief and simple. Be aware that by consciously affirming your wishes, you are invoking powerful spiritual laws to support your life. It is therefore essential to make your affirmations positive. Negative wishes and words should be avoided. For example:

'I am now feeling happy,' instead of, 'I never want to be depressed again.'

'I am now having the most wonderful relationship with the most perfect man for me,' instead of 'I will not become involved with another alcoholic.'

'I am now doing the work I love,' instead of 'I will look for a better job.'

'I am now in perfect health and feel full of energy,' instead of 'I will feel better if I have no more headaches.'

Affirmations will only be effective if used regularly, preferably daily. Nine is said to be the number of completion. Therefore, affirmations are often made nine times or in three groups of three, spaced out during the day. Consciously creating positive affirmations is a pleasurable experience—enjoy it, and the results!

CASE HISTORIES

STEPHANIE

Stephanie felt her life was in a mess. Despite working as a psychic counsellor, she did not have any solutions to her health problems and the rift which had developed in her marriage. She was deeply unhappy that she and her husband no longer appeared to be on the same wavelength. His attitude was moody and often unpleasant. Stephanie could understand his concern over their financial problems, which had arisen from negative equity in their house, his dissatisfaction with work and his direction in life, but was disappointed by his unwillingness to communicate with her. She was also most hurt that the joyous occasion of the birth of her first grandchild (this was her second marriage), had been clouded by his lack of interest. He did not support Stephanie's desire to visit her daughter once a week to help with the baby.

The family budget had been boosted by Stephanie's income from working two nights a week as a care assistant in a nursing home. But with her fiftieth birthday looming, Stephanie was feeling ill and exhausted, resentful at having to go on working and frustrated at not being able to pursue more creative interests. She was seriously considering ending the marriage and striking out on her own.

After years of suffering with PMT and cystitis, Stephanie found her menstrual cycle becoming erratic. She started getting hot flushes two or three times a day. She was also finding it difficult to sleep at night or during the daytime, and would often be woken by violent leg cramps. A dry vagina made intercourse extremely uncomfortable. Dieting had not really addressed the problem of steady weight gain. However, most worrying to her was the deterioration in her mental state. She would regularly plunge into periods of deep gloom for no apparent reason. The depression would last a day or two, then lift as suddenly as it had arrived. She was also finding it a strain to do her counselling work because she had become forgetful and had difficulty in remaining focused on what was being said.

Stephanie compared notes with friends and was a little comforted to learn that many of her symptoms were probably attributable to the menopause. HRT was suggested by Stephanie's doctor and she made a thorough evaluation of the treatment for herself. Its risks and side-effects, coupled with her horror at discovering the cruelty inflicted on pregnant mares in order to make some of the oestrogen products, resulted in her discounting this method of treatment.

Stephanie had belonged to a psychic circle for some years and was delighted when another member, who was also experiencing menopausal problems, offered free counselling and support. They put together their own programmes of self-help. Stephanie's diet consisted mainly of highly processed, quick-to-prepare convenience foods, an excess of dairy products and sugary foods, but was almost devoid of fresh fruit and vegetables. She would drink several cups of coffee during the day and endless cups while on night duty. Even though she had little time for lengthy food preparation, Stephanie was still able to make sweeping changes in her eating habits—she bought organic fruit and vegetables from a local market stall and made nourishing vegetable soups, stir-fries with brown rice, and changed to wholemeal and wholegrain products. She omitted dairy products and tea and coffee from her diet, substituting tofu and nuts for protein, soya milk, filtered and still spring water, herb teas and

Barleycup. She also drastically reduced her sugar intake and began to take vitamin E and Evening Primrose oil in supplement form. Stephanie was thrilled at how swiftly her energy levels rose, and also noticed she was getting less PMT and fewer hot flushes.

Seeing the need for additional exercise, Stephanie began to leave her car at home whenever possible and walked, often using some of this time to make positive affirmations. Although this relaxed her body and mind she felt there was still work to be done. She decided to use meditation in her healing process. Having learnt Transcendental Meditation while she was living in California in the 1960s, and meditating from time to time in her psychic circle, Stephanie was able to work out a personal programme of practice and stick to it—half an hour a day, every day. She used simple breathing techniques and routines to stimulate certain energy centres in the body with a view to balancing and strengthening their associated organs and functions. She worked with colour and visualisations to release and forgive her deeply-held feelings of resentment, guilt and hurt from her unhappy first marriage. Looking ahead, she visualised her present matrimonial differences being resolved and a life including creative enjoyment, not limited by financial or other unwanted obligations.

The ongoing counselling also enabled Stephanie to explore and acknowledge many issues she had neglected over the years and, as her mental and emotional state improved, she found openings to have meaningful discussions with her husband. Solutions were found to many of their problems. An opportunity was presented to them to start a low outlay small business selling antiques, something in which they were both interested. The business took off and Stephanie was able to give up the care work.

A year after starting on her holistic programme Stephanie feels like a new woman—she hasn't had a cold or catarrh, has lost two stones in weight, feels balanced, sleeps well, enjoys sex once again and feels in control of her future.

LAURA

'I'm smothered with eczema and beside myself with the itching. The doctor says it's drug-related,' Laura told a friend whom she knew to be interested in complementary therapies. At fifty-four, with her husband holidaying abroad, she felt abandoned and at a loss to know what to do. The friend suggested applying homoeopathic Calendula cream for the itching, taking Evening Primrose oil, and cutting down on meat, dairy products and foods containing processed oils. She enquired what drugs Laura had been taking. 'Nothing for years, other than HRT,' she said. 'The doctor has now shown me a list of possible side-effects. I never would have taken it if I had known.'

Laura was the eldest of six children. The family were working class and poor. After their mother was widowed, Laura was expected to look after her younger brothers and sisters. One of her earliest memories was being sent to the pawn shop.

Marrying late, she gave birth to her only child at forty. Her husband quietly controlled the relationship. Considered to be at the top of his profession, his high earning power enabled them to travel regularly to France to sample its gastronomic delights. They also enjoyed rich food and good wine at home. Laura was in awe of her husband and put huge effort into the marriage and home. Life revolved around him, their son, and entertaining a procession of house guests. The marriage had been happy, the only rift occurring when Laura's mother-in-law came to live with them shortly before she died.

Menopause had produced no drastic symptoms for Laura—every now and again her eyelids would become sore and swell up for a few days; her digestion sometimes reacted to the rich food; and her skin felt dry and had begun to sag in places. Rather more serious for her was that her slight loss of libido had been noticed by her husband, who was a sexually demanding man. It was probably the fear of his being unfaithful which prompted Laura to request HRT, an action which was encouraged by her husband who openly enjoyed having an attractive, much younger wife. Laura joked, 'He wants me to look like Joan Collins for ever.'

At around this time, a woman friend and her terminally ill husband came to stay. Laura pulled out all the stops to make the sick man's stay comfortable and happy. She had never felt entirely comfortable in his presence before, but on this occasion, the last time she was to see him before his death shortly afterwards, they talked in great depth. A loving bond formed between them. Laura felt highly valued and that she had something to offer him. This incident, his death and the feelings surrounding her eczema problem triggered off a new awareness in Laura. She took steps to use it for positive change and healing.

Laura consulted a homoeopath about her eczema and was given a remedy which cleared the condition. She enrolled in a daytime yoga class at which the teacher suggested specific postures to help Laura. Some of the women in the class also attended a weekly meditation and study group which Laura joined. It took a few weeks before she felt she was meditating successfully, but Laura persevered, practising at home nearly every day. Meditation proved to be an inner pathway to self-discovery and transformation for Laura. With the help of the group leader, she first worked on releasing deeply held fears and her need to please people, which she related to issues concerning withdrawal of affection. She was also able to release suppressed and more recent grief.

Laura observed the emergence of hidden qualities and strengths. She became more clear about her needs, developing the confidence to express them. She was able to talk to her husband about their relationship and tell him how she felt about her sexuality. Laura's future marital role was clarified, to their mutual satisfaction. Physical changes also occurred. Her skin tone improved and she felt more energetic, not needing a nap after lunch. Laura enthuses about the benefits of meditation. She has continued to practise and is now taking a correspondence course in nutrition.

KATE

Kate was struggling through a disastrous menopause when her life fell apart. Her husband died suddenly from a heart attack, leaving her at the age of fifty well provided for but with two children of eleven and fourteen to bring up alone. She was on sick leave from the firm of accountants where she had worked throughout her marriage and felt far from being able to return. The severity of her menopausal mood swings had increased since her bereavement. Her mind swung like a pendulum. One moment she would plunge into helpless despair, clinging to the children and her memories. The next might bring an outburst of anger which frightened them all.

Normally a capable, contained person, Kate was difficult

to get close to, but not unreasonable. She had fallen into a state of denial, refusing to acknowledge or discuss problems. Kate's menopausal problems had started when was forty-eight. After suffering appalling night sweats, exhaustion and stress incontinence, she went to her doctor with a request for HRT. She put up with minor side-effects, taking the treatment on and off for two years, when brown patches started to appear on her arms then neck. The doctor thought this was a side-effect of HRT. Kate tried the treatment once more, but gave up altogether when the patches worsened. In addition to the original symptoms, which were still in evidence, she now found herself waking in the night having panic attacks.

Kate attempted to relieve her tension, choosing to workout at a gym and at home, but found the programme of exercise too strenuous. She became very thin and even more dejected. Her mind felt scrambled. A friend at the gym suggested the more gentle relaxation measures of listening to music and keep-fit classes. Kate took these on board, finding that the music gave her a degree of solace and peace. The friend also recommended meditation for healing and clearing the mind, lending Kate a beginners' guide. The first beneficial change she noticed, after a period of quietly working at home by the book, was a lessening of tension and the disappearance of indigestion pains round the heart. Greatly relieved, she bought a book on healing using meditation and visualisation techniques, finding more guidance from a short course in meditation and colour healing.

Kate's personal meditation and visualisation programme included working with symbols and colour. She used green (balances, harmonises—helps the nervous system) in open-air scenes; blue for peace and healing and a river scene in which she sat on the bank with her feet in the water.

(Visualisations involving water are important for negative thoughts such as bitterness and frustration. To have the feet in water is very healing and useful in release work.)

Kate was able gently to release her pent-up grief. Sometimes during periods when her mind was totally quiet she was comforted and guided by a calm voice within. Not only was she becoming stronger on the outside, but she felt that she was gaining greater strength on the inside. Her night sweats and panic attacks subsided within three months and the stress incontinence did not occur so frequently. As time went on, Kate found coping much easier. People noticed how her personality had changed—becoming softer, more flexible.

Kate took one year off work. Towards the end of this time she decided to seek the help of a bereavement counsellor and derived much benefit from the sessions. Meditation brought Kate to a point of clarity, balance and peace.

CHAPTER THIRTEEN

Nutrition and Diet

Let food be your medicine
Hippocrates

Dietary therapy in one form or another is one of the most ancient known methods of healing and has been practised in different ways in virtually every culture throughout the world. Modern nutritional therapy has developed out of increasing scientific research this century into vitamins, minerals and their relationship to health, and from the clinical ecology, allergy and environmental medicine movement of the 1940s. This research has been combined with traditional naturopathic principles to form nutritional therapy as we know it today.

WHAT IS NUTRITIONAL THERAPY?
Nutritional therapy involves working with a trained and qualified practitioner. It includes a diagnostic procedure and a prescription that will involve dietary advice, supplements, medicinal herbs, naturopathic techniques, detoxification, lifestyle and exercise recommendations, as well as other suggestions depending upon individual needs. Practitioners are usually trained over at least three years; training includes the medical sciences as well as naturopathic and environmental principles related to health. In more general terms, nutritional therapy could also include any procedure that involves the therapeutic use of nutrition.

A nutritional therapist works differently from a

conventional dietitian or nutritionist practising along medical lines. Normally, hospital or other dietitians give advice upon the recommendations and diagnosis of a medical doctor. This approach attempts to treat the results of a condition—for instance, obesity related to excessive calorie intake—rather than the deeper nutritional or other causes which a nutritional therapist would consider.

NUTRITIONAL THERAPY AND MENOPAUSE

In nutritional therapy (NT), menopause is not looked upon as an illness, but as a perfectly natural occurrence in a woman's life. It is simply the end of one long hormonal cycle that started at puberty and the fact that some women suffer more than others must be attributable to natural and understandable reasons. NT helps by looking for and understanding the nutritional causes for the problems that some women suffer, reasoning that once discovered, they can usually be helped.

Nature is full of cycles and cycles are concerned with the process of change. Changes that occur in all forms of nature, including the human menopause, can only go well if the right supply of nourishment or raw materials are available and things are working in a balanced and optimal way. Nutritional therapy provides the raw materials and other strategies that help make menopause an easy phase.

A useful analogy is to look at your body as a building you inhabit through the three main cycles of life: childhood, adulthood and old age. The first cycle of childhood is one of growth, when your building is still being constructed; the second cycle is adult life when your building is being used for work; the third cycle is when your building should increasingly be used as a comfortable retirement home. The transition between the second and third cycles is the menopause, when your building has to be converted to your retirement home. However, if there is a lack of sound building materials (nutritional raw materials) when it comes to converting the building, it won't be possible to do a good job. In fact, most of the symptoms of menopause problems can be understood if you realise they are due to the body trying to do a job of conversion whilst in a depleted state.

NUTRITIONAL PREVENTION AND TREATMENT OF MENOPAUSAL SYMPTOMS

We all know that prevention is easier than cure, so the simple fact is that the best way to have an easy menopause and avoid taking HRT is to get into a good nutritional state and general good health for as long as possible before it starts. This does not mean that problems cannot be helped once the menopause begins, but it does mean that you will have more to do if you leave it until then. Nutritional prevention is a good investment and just as sensible as a pension or insurance policy. The nutritional causes of the problems that occur in the menopause can broadly be divided into two main categories:

1. Lack of positive nutrition in the diet before menopause.
2. Excess of anti-nutritional factors in the diet before menopause.

The main problem with dietary habits in the developed world is not one of quantity or availability, but of nutritional quality. Many women eat an adequate amount of vitamins, minerals, fibre, protein, carbohydrate and the other essential nutrients. However, the anti-nutritional factors in their diet often outweigh the positive ones, and create a slow hidden depletion. Anti-nutritional factors tend to be products consumed that have very little nutritional value but which, at the same time, deplete the body further. The most common are: tea; coffee; added sugar (sucrose); excessive alcohol; chocolate; added refined salt or sodium products; for example MSG (monosodium glutamate); refined foods such as white flour products; artificial additives (many of the E additives); over-cooking and over-use of pre-cooked or convenience foods.

There is no such thing as one good diet that is suitable for all. However, there are certain types of foods that are bad and others that are good for just about everyone. The Good Food Guide that follows indicates the mainly positive nutritional factors needed for the menopause, as well as anti-nutritional items to avoid in the diet.

GOOD FOOD GUIDE FOR THE MENOPAUSE
Organics
General Recommendation Avoid non-organic food whenever possible. Choose organic produce, or be sure to peel non-organic produce. The residues of artificial chemicals in non-organic foods are related to a growing number of health problems, including hormonal ones. It is quite possible that these residues are contributing to your menopausal problems and may lead to more difficulties in the future. Organic food is safer, more nutritious—and it tastes better.

Fluids
Generally Good Pure water, such as spring water (non-carbonated), filtered water, water that has been boiled for fifteen minutes, herbal teas, coffee substitutes, e.g. Barleycup,

Yannoh, Caro, dandelion coffee, vegetable and fruit juices.

Menopause is often made worse by dehydration on a cellular level (not dehydration in the normal sense), which makes it hard for the body to detoxify, balance and restore itself. Cellular dehydration is due to drinking mainly diuretics, such as tea, coffee and alcohol; not having enough pure water; and eating too much salt. The body also tends to recognise all fluids except water as foods, and so uses them differently from water.

Generally Bad Ordinary tea, coffee, alcohol, chilled drinks. These generally increase hot flushes. Not only do these drinks lack goodness, but they leach out important nutrients from the body and hinder absorption from food. Chilled drinks reduce digestive ability and absorption. See also above.

General Recommendations Drink more water (particularly hot), minimum one pint a day, preferably two to four pints a day. Cut out coffee and tea (or reduce tea to about two cups a day). It is better to have unchilled drinks if you have digestive or absorption problems. Have more herbal teas, coffee alternatives and vegetable and fruit juices. Organic juice can be purchased from health food shops or specialist companies.

Grains
Grains include cereals, flours, pasta, breads or bakery products, and most forms of starchy foods or carbohydrates. Any woman approaching or in her menopause should reduce or avoid wheat, wheat flour, pasta and bakery products made from wheat flour, in particular white flour.

Wheat is no longer the 'staff of life' it used to be. Modern varieties are hybrids that are much more reliant upon artificial chemicals. Wheat has a much higher level of gluten than any other grain, which makes it harder to digest. It is also a very common allergen.

Who benefits from avoiding wheat or white flour? Usually anyone with digestive and bowel problems, weight problems, allergy symptoms, candida, fatigue and menopausal problems.

General Recommendations Eat less wheat and avoid white flour completely. All other grains and flours are usually better, especially whole rice, oat flakes and flour, rye bread, barley flour, non-wheat pasta. Choose organic wholemeal flour if you use wheat at all.

Vegetables

General Recommendations Almost all vegetables are very good for you and most people benefit from increasing the amount and variety of them in their diet. Vegetables are nature's multi-vitamins. You get a wide range of vitamins if you have about five different vegetables with your main meals. Mix different colours as well as varieties that are grown above and below ground. Tinned or frozen vegetables have much less goodness than fresh ones, so eat fresh whenever possible. Do not overcook. Try and use the water in which the vegetables are cooked, for instance as stock or in a sauce, as there is much goodness left in it.

Not So Good Vegetables of the deadly nightshade family—e.g. tomatoes, potatoes, peppers and aubergines—should be eaten less often than other vegetables.

Cooked tomatoes (tinned, purée, sauces/ketchup, etc.) are acidic and best avoided in people with skin conditions, arthritis, hot flushes and liver problems. Tomatoes are also a common allergen. Potatoes are more toxic if sprouting or green and are also generally bad for those with depression. Eat these vegetables in moderation, generally not more than twice a week.

Fruit

General Recommendation Most fruits are fine in moderation, but they tend to cause more problems than vegetables. As a general rule, eat a lot more vegetables and less fruit. Oranges can cause problems for many people, as can, to a lesser extent, other citrus fruits such as satsumas, tangerines, grapefruit, lemon, lime and pineapples.

Fruit tends to stimulate the release of toxins from the tissues or organs of the body. This is a good thing, but quite often the body cannot cope with an excessive overload on its channels of elimination, such as the bowel and kidneys. The net result may be an aggravation of symptoms. People often experience this when doing a fruit fast.

Legumes or Pulses

This category includes all dried beans, peas, lentils and most soya products.

General Recommendations Most people can benefit from having more pulses and less animal protein. Pulses are rich in fibre and have no harmful fats. When mixed with grains (e.g. beans on toast or lentils and rice), they form a complete protein and so provide an alternative to animal sources of protein. Most pulses, with the exception of red lentils, require soaking in water for several hours (preferably overnight) prior to long cooking until tender.

Note Dried pulses should be boiled for at least ten minutes before reducing the heat and simmering for the required time.

Nuts

General Recommendations Most nuts are fine in moderation, the main exception being peanuts (groundnuts, or monkey nuts), which can be extremely dangerous to people who are allergic to them. Nuts are best eaten fresh from the shell. Almonds are particularly good. If you are trying to lose weight or experiencing liver problems, keep nuts to a minimum and use seeds instead.

Seeds

These include sunflower, pumpkin, sesame, flax or linseeds.

General Recommendations Seeds are very good for most people — they can be eaten in greater quantity than nuts and are lower in fats. Seeds are rich in proteins and often in minerals, e.g. pumpkin seeds are a rich source of zinc, and sesame of calcium. Some have beneficial oils, such as flax or linseeds, which are rich in Omega 3 and Omega 6 EFAs (essential fatty acids). Sunflower spread is a good alternative to peanut butter, as is sesame cream (or tahini), which has as much calcium per pound as Cheddar cheese.

Seeds can be purchased ready sprouted, or sprouting can easily be done at home. Sprouted seeds, which retain all their nutrients and develop more beneficial properties, are excellent in salads.

Note Linseeds should be soaked for a few hours before eating. Add 5 fl oz water to two teaspoonfuls of linseeds for daily use.

Fats and Oils

These include vegetable oils, margarines, animal fats.

Generally Good In moderation, olive oil and unheated vegetable (polyunsaturated) oils, especially linseed or flax seed oil. Cold-pressed oils are best. Small amounts of non-hydrogenated margarines and small amounts of animal fats; especially clarified butter or ghee, are fine.

Generally Bad Heated vegetable oils (except olive oil), ordinary hydrogenated margarines. Animal fats in anything but very small amounts.

Most vegetable oils, or polyunsaturates, are damaged by heat. This creates platelet aggregation in the blood which may, as with saturated fats, lead to heart disease. Most oils used in the manufacture of ordinary margarines are similarly damaged when hydrogen is pumped through them to harden them (these are known as hydrogenated oils). The result may be the hardening of the cell walls in the body and lead to immune system problems.

General Recommendations Women with 'dry' menopause conditions such as dry vagina, dry skin and joint problems benefit the most from a moderate intake of the right oils and fats. Those with hot flushes, fibrocystic conditions or excess weight, however, should minimise all oils and fats in the diet (except Omega 3 and Omega 6 GLAs). If cooking, use only olive or clarified butter.

Note Excess fat (and protein) in the diet may contribute to bone loss.

Sweet Foods

Generally Good In moderation, most natural sweeteners such as fruits, fruit juice concentrates, fruit sugar (fructose), natural honey (untreated), maple syrup, molasses, jaggery (a natural sugar obtainable in ethnic areas), barley malt and brown rice syrup.

Generally Bad Ordinary white or brown sugar (sucrose), sugar syrups (e.g. golden syrup), glucose, dextrose, artificial sweeteners, heat-treated or cooked honey. Too much honey or molasses can increase hot flushes.

Recommendations The more concentrated the sweetness in a food, the less you should have at any one time; for instance, you could have a larger portion of fruit than honey. For weight loss, minimise sweet foods and use honey, molasses and, in particular, jaggery.

Condiments

Generally Good Mild and natural spices, herbs, sauces or chutney.

Generally Bad Salt and any sauces, ketchups or chutneys that are heavily laced with salt or ordinary sugar.

We nearly all have an excess of salt in our bodies that has built up over many years. In nature, salt (sodium) is rare, so the body is designed to conserve it, whereas other minerals such as magnesium and potassium are excreted easily. Salt consumption has increased enormously in modern times. Excess salt displaces magnesium and potassium, locks up calcium, making it unavailable for use and contributes to many health problems. Also avoid baking soda, bicarbonate of soda, sodium bicarbonate and monosodium glutamate (MSG).

Recommendations Use many more herbs and spices in your cooking. They not only have a much wider range of tastes than salt, but also have positive medicinal effects, helping digestion and the absorption of goodness from foods. If you have hot flushes, avoid very hot spices such as cayenne or chilli. Reduce salt slowly over about two weeks—most people find that after a month they enjoy the taste of food much more without it. Salt substitutes based upon potassium can be used in small amounts.

Animal Products
Generally Good Meat eaten in moderation. People with depletion and menopause problems can benefit from some animal products, in particular organic, low-fat, free-range produce such as chicken, turkey, rabbit, venison, ostrich and game.
Generally Bad Non-organic, high in fat and red meat is harmful for most people, especially those with hot flushes or excess weight. Products to be avoided include beef, pork, ham, bacon, lamb or similar types of meat and meat products, e.g. sausages, burgers, pâté and mince.

Fish and Seafood
Generally Good Most fish is better than meat if from unpolluted waters. Edible seaweeds are also very nutritious, if you can acquire a taste for them.
Generally Bad Fish that is highly salted, tinned or smoked, shellfish and polluted fish.

Dairy Produce and Eggs
Generally Good Some in moderation, and better if organic and low fat. Products made from goat's or sheep's milk are less commonly allergenic than those made from cow's milk.
Generally Bad Non-organic, high-fat produce, hard cheese (especially if cooked), mouldy cheeses. Dairy products are common allergens and are a problem for many people, especially those with catarrhal or weight problems.
Note All dairy products are acid-forming.

GENERAL DIETARY RECOMMENDATIONS
Eat fewer animal products generally, have more vegetable proteins (pulses combined with grains/cereals, etc.). As a

general guide, consume foods in the following proportions per week:

meat—once or twice

fish—two or three times

eggs—not more than two

low-fat yoghurt—a little most days

cottage cheese or other low-fat cheese (goat's/ewe's)—twice.

Alternatives Rice milk, soya milk and other soya products can be used or if you have an allergy to animal products.

MAGNESIUM AND CALCIUM

Most people believe that calcium is the main nutrient to supplement at menopause. However, recent research indicates that for the adequate metabolism or utilisation of calcium in the body there is actually a need for more magnesium than calcium.

Magnesium is the co-catalyst for more enzymes in the body than any other mineral. Practically nothing happens in the body that is not related in one way or another to magnesium. Magnesium is found in a wide variety of foods—whole grains, fresh vegetables (particularly greens), pulses, fresh fruit. When it is established that there is a deficiency of magnesium in the individual, supplementation is known to help many physical and mental health problems, including osteoporosis, joint and muscle pain, pre-menstrual tension, insomnia, depression and tiredness.

HOW TO CHANGE TO YOUR NEW DIET

Make the easiest changes to your existing diet first. Read through the Good Food Guide and make notes about your responses to the information in it. If you find yourself resisting the idea of reducing certain items, reduce those items gradually or leave them until later. Only make about fifty per cent of the recommended changes to your diet during the first week.

DEALING WITH ADDICTIONS AND CRAVINGS

You may be coming off addictive foods and drinks and experience withdrawal symptoms. If these are severe, then indulge a little to relieve the symptoms, but generally reduce them until you can do without completely. Like withdrawal from any addiction, the symptoms pass if you stick at it and you are left feeling much better than before.

This specialised dietary advice is unlikely to be appropriate for the rest of your life. It is designed to help your body to nourish and re-balance itself through the menopause. For more specialised individual advice you should consult a nutritional therapist.

CASE HISTORIES

CAROLINE

Caroline, aged fifty, a busy and successful massage therapist with one grown-up son, attended her first consultation with a nutritional therapist complaining of the following symptoms, which had been increasing over the past year: headaches, hot flushes and night sweats, feeling stressed and anxious, finding it difficult to cope, low energy, also stress incontinence and bloating of the abdomen. No conventional or other medicines were being taken.

The Nutritional Diagnosis

Low in B vitamins generally, especially B6, also low in vitamins C and D, lacking in high quality essential fatty acids (Omega 3 and 6), low in chromium, magnesium and calcium.

Caroline was generally depleted, tense, nervous, run down, had a poorly functioning liver and a sluggish bowel. The therapist prescribed linseeds and more water for the bowel (linseeds are also rich in essential fatty acids), plus aloe vera juice for the bowel and liver, along with lecithin for the liver and nervous system.

The diet recommended was along the lines in this chapter, but with an emphasis on foods to help restore, ground and calm, as well as focusing on the liver.

At her second consultation, Caroline was not much better, but things were beginning to change: her bowel function was improving, she felt more calm, less anxious and was generally functioning in a more balanced way. She had also become aware of how stressful situations and overwork increased her flushing symptoms. In addition to her original prescription, the therapist introduced B complex, vitamin C and magnesium supplements and reduced the level of lecithin. Herbs were also recommended to be taken.

After another four weeks of treatment, at her next consultation Caroline reported feeling much better generally, in particular more emotionally stable. Her flushing was minimal, she had far fewer headaches and was feeling more positive and able to be assertive in relationships and dealings with others.

Caroline decided to continue with the diet and supporting treatment as she was continually moving in and out of stressful situations or working excessively hard. She had come to recognise her life pattern for her, of a decline in her health every time she was confronted with these circumstances. She began to seek more permanent solutions, creating greater balance in her life and gradually needing less help.

Conclusion

This case is a good example of a health or nutritional spending and saving situation. In simple terms, this meant that the patient felt improvement from her recommended nutritional therapy (saving or input), and then repeated a long-term pattern of overdoing things and getting into highly stressful situations (over-spending or recreating a nutritional overdraft). Gradually, however, the nutritional therapy gave Caroline the support she needed to help her recognise the pattern and the awareness to change it.

ROSEMARY

Rosemary, a teacher with two grown-up daughters, was fifty when she consulted a nutritional therapist. Symptoms noted at her first consultation were: hot flushes, panic attacks, lack of energy, insomnia, feeling a lack of purpose in life, depression, weak capillaries in the fingers, hay fever and migraine, aching knees, elbows and finger joints, sinusitis and dry, itchy skin patches. She was not taking any medication, apart from occasional painkillers for migraine.

The Nutritional Diagnosis

The diagnosis showed up the effects of stress and blood sugar problems (hypoglycaemia) and lowered immune function. Nutritionally, Rosemary was low in just about every possible nutrient, even though she had been taking a selection of supplements for some time (an indication that either her digestion/absorption was poor, or the form of supplements taken were of poor quality). She was depleted and had poor liver function (a common combination in menopausal problems) as well as some bowel sluggishness. Firstly, dietary improvements were recommended, together with aloe vera juice, plus alkaline vitamin C with extra bioflavenoids (to help the capillaries and circulation, as well as the bowel and liver). Some herbs were also given to help balance and clear her system generally. It was recommended that she gradually come off her current supplements.

Three weeks later, at Rosemary's next consultation, her system was clearer, so new supplements, rich in B vitamins and minerals and easy to absorb and metabolise, were introduced.

In her next report, after a further three weeks, Rosemary said her flushes had eased, she had more energy, her sleep had improved and she was more able to cope emotionally. She had also come to realise that emotional blocks had been preventing progress, but now felt more inclined to tackle this. The therapist suggested she might seek counselling or psychotherapy if she felt comfortable with this idea.

Rosemary's symptoms continued to improve and, after another three weeks, she reported having more energy; the flushing and panic attacks were eighty per cent better, sleep seventy per cent better; positivity and feelings about lack of purpose in life fifty per cent better. The hay fever season was underway, but Rosemary's symptoms only developed if she was in a grassy area. In addition to the other treatments, she was given vitamin B5 and chromium to help her hypoglycaemia and boost her adrenal function, thus increasing energy levels.

A month later, Rosemary reported less flushing, she was

sleeping well, had no headaches and felt more balanced emotionally. She continued the treatment and, after a further month, reported that she was feeling more energetic. Her capillaries and all other symptoms were greatly improved. It was recommended that she continue treatment for another three months.

Rosemary returned to the therapist seven months later having had a depressing winter. She had mostly let the previous recommendations slip and had been off the treatment a long time. Her condition was re-assessed and showed that she had become somewhat congested and toxic, but her condition had not completely reverted. The therapist prescribed some cleansing and detoxification of the liver (liver congestion was causing depression) and gentle cleansing of the body generally, mainly through dietary changes, simple herbs and additional vitamin C. She was also asked, one day a week, to have a liquid-only day, during which she could eat as much as she liked, but in a liquid form—a simple, gentle fast. In addition, she took extra B complex and additional B5 and rutin. From this point on, she needed less treatment.

Conclusion

This patient was progressing well until a long gap was left between consultations. This was combined with a change in seasons, which brought changes in her diet and metabolism. This combination of factors created a situation where she let the treatment slip and gradually became more congested. Many of her old symptoms returned (primarily depression). Rosemary's case highlights how a seasonal change can affect some women, and can often warrant a review in diagnosis and treatment. Rosemary experienced, as do many people, an increased awareness of and desire to deal with emotional issues in her life once she was more nutritionally and physically supported and balanced.

MACROBIOTICS
A Return to Nature Can Heal
WHAT IS MACROBIOTICS?

The macrobiotic way of life recognises that there is a natural order of the universe. It embraces the simple principles of respecting the cycles of nature, living with sensitivity to and in harmony with ourselves, the universal life force and the environment of which we are an integral part. This way of life has always been with us and continues to be lived naturally all over the world among traditional peoples.

At the heart of this broader philosophy lies the macrobiotic way of eating. Although its popularity as a method of healing a wide range of symptoms continues to grow, public awareness is still scant. It has unfairly gained the reputation of being a disciplined, narrow and restrictive way of eating. In fact, the macrobiotic diet offers a firm foundation for good health. Its philosophy is to eat, simply and naturally, traditional, whole, unrefined foods, primarily locally grown; cooked appropriately for each season and in tune with the weather conditions.

The original macrobiotic diet was created by a Japanese scholar, George Ohsawa, who died in 1966. When still in his teens, he was told by orthodox doctors that he was dying from tuberculosis and had only a few months to live. George Ohsawa refused to accept this prognosis. He proceeded to study Eastern medicine and philosophy, developing a style of eating which followed the underlying principles of the Eastern approach to life and using traditional local food. In adhering to these principles, he healed himself.

Introducing more wholesome foods into your larder does not have to be put in hand all at once. Having made the initial outlay on the basics, other ingredients can be bought as required, according to the speed at which you are progressing. Macrobiotics has incorrectly gained the reputation of being an expensive way of eating. Weigh the cost of whole, natural/organic foods against meat, convenience/processed foods, vitamin supplements and even the cost of medicine—or being unwell!

MACROBIOTIC DIETARY TREATMENT OF MENOPAUSE SYMPTOMS

As menopause draws near, there are tremendous benefits to be gained from changing your diet and adopting a more vegetarian, natural approach. To start making changes when you are much younger is better still. Eating animal foods tends to overheat the body, loading the system with unwanted excesses. The ending of menstruation also sees the ending of a very important process of discharge and elimination. The body may then find it difficult to get rid of accumulated excesses and toxins. The metabolism slows down generally and is very different from the high-performance body you had as a twenty-year-old.

Saturated fats—animal foods such as meats, dairy products and eggs— are stored in the body, especially in a woman's reproductive system, producing stagnation and accumulation. These may cause hot flushes/night sweats, excessive bleeding, fibroids (gathering of fats), water retention, varicose veins, stiffness and irritability. The body, therefore, needs to find ways to eliminate and discharge them.

By contrast, an excess of products such as sugar, chocolate, ice-cream and alcohol often create symptoms such as vertigo, itching skin, leg cramps, fatigue, mood swings, depression, lack of concentration and osteoporosis.

Many menopausal symptoms could be prevented or considerably alleviated by stabilising eating habits, aiming towards a natural diet, in order to achieve balance and well-being. The rainbow of symptoms cannot, however, be separated and cured one by one. The human being is a unity—everything affects the balance of the whole. Using food as an 'aspirin' for these or any other symptoms will not work if the whole person is not embraced. Overall, the message is to eat in a well-balanced way, then everything will normalise.

Chewing

Chewing is the first step in activating the digestive process. The action of chewing produces saliva which contains a digestive enzyme responsible for breaking down complex carbohydrates into sugars, then glucose. If food is not chewed properly, this enzyme does not reach the intestines. They are then put under strain, the acid balance is upset and feelings of discomfort and flatulence may result. Proper, unhurried chewing is relaxing and not only improves the taste of food and prevents over-eating, but activates many other organs and functions in the body which protect against disease.

Chewing produces a hormone in the saliva which strengthens teeth and gums and another hormone, parotin, which stimulates cell metabolism, regenerates the body and keeps it looking young. Wholefoods such as beans, grains and vegetables, should be chewed properly for their beneficial effects throughout the whole body.

Dietary Guidelines

Changing your dietary habits and eating within macrobiotic guidelines can bring feelings of greater balance, sensitivity and often a different view of reality. The health benefits are enormous: relief or complete recovery from illness of all types from weight problems, acne and eczema to PMS and menopausal symptoms.

A TYPICAL MACROBIOTIC DIET

A typical macrobiotic diet includes daily portions of: wholegrains and grain products; seasonal vegetables; beans; vegetarian proteins; fish; seafood and sea vegetables; fermented foods, e.g. soya sauce, sauerkraut (to help digestion and promote healthy intestinal flora); soup to which miso (fermented soya bean/grain curd, obtainable from health food stores) is often added; local and seasonal fruits; natural sweeteners and puddings; seeds; nuts; and healthy snacks.

Use a variety of ingredients, select a variety of cooking styles and try to create simple recipes. Planning and organisation will reduce time spent in the kitchen.

Sea Vegetables

Sea vegetables, thoughtfully prepared, are often used in macrobiotic cooking. For centuries, people all over the world have harvested sea vegetables for use as food. In the British Isles, our best-known sea vegetable dish is the traditional Welsh laver bread (laver and oats). In Scotland, dulse is served in oat porridge. Sea vegetables are among the most nutritious foods on earth, containing a host of vitamins, minerals and trace elements, often lacking in vegetables grown on land in soil depleted by chemical fertilisers.

Sea vegetables from the brown algae family include kombu, wakame, arame and hijiki. Wakame is invaluable to women—it nourishes the reproductive organs, helps to regulate the menstrual cycle and improves the condition of the skin and hair. Kombu nourishes the adrenals and kidneys in addition to helping the reproductive organs.

Puddings and Sweeteners

You can still enjoy sweet puddings, fruit pies, jellies, cakes and spreads on a macrobiotic diet, using natural ingredients. These include fresh and dried fruits, seeds, nuts, natural sweeteners, citric peel, cinnamon, vanilla, carob, ginger, nutmeg, ground almonds, chestnut purée, tahini and rolled oats. Try using soya yoghurts and desserts, sweets made from natural ingredients, cereal bars, natural fruit juices, natural fruit jams, a natural grain-based sweetener such as traditional barley malt extract, corn and barley malt, rice syrup and amasake (a creamy, sweet-tasting dessert/drink made from cultured grain). They are all available from health food shops.

BALANCED MENU IDEAS FOR THE SEASONS
Spring
Breakfast Sweet rice porridge with amasake topping. Roasted sesame seeds. Grain coffee or bancha tea.

Lunch Carrot and orange soup. Vegetable burger in a wholemeal roll with lettuce, cucumber, bean sprouts. Pickles (fermented type, e.g. sauerkraut). Apple.

Supper Quinoa (grain) and sweet corn. Curried tofu with almonds. Crunchy watercress salad. Carrot and green bean salad. Pickles. Lemon mousse.

Summer

Breakfast Stewed apples Wholemeal bread with peanut butter spread. Grain coffee.

Lunch Couscous salad (with chickpeas, vegetables, seeds). Pressed salad—cucumber, radish, celery. Pickles. Carrot/apple juice.

Supper Tagliatelle with home-made pesto sauce. Mediterranean green salad (with wakame, olives and vegetables). Fish and vegetable kebabs with barbecue sauce. Pickles. Summer berry trifle.

Autumn

Breakfast Scrambled tofu on toast. Blanched watercress. Grain coffee.

Lunch Chunky vegetable soup with wholemeal garlic bread. Bean pâté. Celery sticks. Pickles. Grain coffee made with rice milk.

Supper Minestrone soup with millet and vegetables. Fish pie. Green salad with vinaigrette. Steamed vegetables with tofu dressing. Steamed pears with carob and hazelnut sauce. Herb tea.

Winter

Breakfast Creamy porridge oats with roasted sunflower seeds. Boiled carrot slices. Grain cinnamon coffee.

Lunch Wholemeal bread sandwiches with smoked tofu and salad with sauerkraut. Nut mix (nuts and dried fruit). Steamed vegetables. Sweet ginger tea.

Supper Stir-fried vegetables and pasta with sesame seeds and ginger. Lentil loaf/roast. Home-made coleslaw with tofu mayonnaise. Boiled kale and Brussels sprouts. Pickles. Baked apple.

CASE HISTORIES

LUCY

Lucy, a forty-nine-year-old-secretary, was already seeing a macrobiotic dietary counsellor when she developed a range of debilitating menopausal symptoms. Pleased with the progress she had made so far, she decided to decline the offer of surgery to deal with a large fibroid and to continue under the care of this practitioner.

Six months previously, Lucy had visited a chiropractor, complaining of severe back pain. Having confirmed that her back was properly aligned, he recommended a macrobiotic counsellor. The counsellor felt that the pain was due to a condition of stress/imbalance of the kidneys. She felt that a long-standing problem Lucy had with her ears—itching and running, necessitating regular syringing—was linked to her kidneys. The practitioner also observed that Lucy was very tense, a fact to which Lucy herself would not readily admit.

Lucy had a history of heavy smoking, alcohol abuse and excess consumption of dairy products. She was no longer smoking and had curtailed her alcohol intake, but she told the counsellor she loved cheese, gold top milk, Greek yoghurt, egg sandwiches, toast and Marmite. She would nibble hard cheese prior to menstruation, believing it would increase her calcium levels. Her menstrual cycle had begun to shorten, but was not giving cause for concern.

A diet was formulated to help regenerate her kidneys and cleanse her body of the accumulated effects of eggs and dairy products. It was recommended that meat, dairy products, eggs, sugar in any form, alcohol, yeast and Marmite be avoided. The new diet contained grains, an abundance of vegetables, sea vegetables and fruit. Protein was provided by beans, soya products, fish and nuts. A large bowl of carrot purée and a bowl of miso vegetable soup was eaten daily. Emphasis was placed on aduki beans—Lucy was also recommended to drink the cooking water. (Aduki tea is useful in helping to adjust kidney imbalance and to release excess water from the body.) Tea and coffee were given up, replaced by bancha tea, grain coffee and herbal teas. Although she found the taste of bancha tea a little strange at first, Lucy soon came to prefer it to ordinary tea. Grain coffees were not a problem.

The counsellor also treated Lucy's back with hot ginger compresses. A ginger compress stimulates blood circulation. The heat and the penetrating quality of the ginger help loosen and dissolve hardened, stagnated accumulations. Lucy's pain subsided and her ear condition improved. Progress was monitored on a monthly basis and seemed to be going well until a stressful period in Lucy's personal life—her mother's illness, problems with her nine-year-old son, relationship difficulties and additional work pressure—heralded a decline in her physical state. Lucy also noticed a significant increase in menstrual bleeding and soreness and discomfort in her abdomen.

A medical examination revealed a large fibroid, the size of a cricket ball. Homoeopathy offered on the NHS helped, but Lucy was told the only sure way to stop the bleeding quickly was to take synthetic progesterone. Lucy was reluctant to continue with this treatment. Other symptoms at the time were: extreme fatigue, depression, candida, a small patch of eczema on the face, hot flushes, stress incontinence, irritability, tension, lack of concentration, poor memory, flatulence, tooth/gum infection (her dentist advised that the gums were receding—a common problem at Lucy's time of life), unsightly swelling (lasting a few days at a time) of the top eyelids.

The macrobiotic counsellor explained that a fibroid was merely a collection of fat. It had taken many years to accumulate and was a result of past extreme eating patterns—too much alcohol, dairy products, eggs, salty food and a lack of fibre and vegetables.

Lucy's diet was duly adjusted and strictly adhered to, with monitoring taking place each week. Oil was reduced to a minimum, and no nuts or peanut butter were permitted— bread was omitted (it does not help accumulations in the reproductive system), as were a lot of raw fruits, which can have a cooling effect, freezing existing fats. Cooked fruits were recommended instead.

To counteract the weakness from blood loss, hijiki sea vegetable was eaten every day. Mineral supplements were also taken and Lucy was encouraged to ensure she had adequate rest and peace. Her practitioner steered her to an emotional counsellor where, over the course of several sessions, many deep-seated issues came to the surface for consideration and release.

Lucy went to her GP for an examination six months later and was delighted to be told that the fibroid had halved in size. She attended a cookery course facilitated by her macrobiotic practitioner, where she gained information that enabled her to design attractive menus for herself. As she had been extremely weak, the practitioner felt that Lucy would also benefit from a herbal tonic, which was obtained after a consultation with a herbalist.

Over the course of the next few months, Lucy's energy levels continued to rise. Her mental state calmed. Menstruation normalised; her cycle lengthened. Other symptoms were considerably relieved or disappeared altogether. Lucy had a further medical check after another six months and was told that the fibroid was now so small it was difficult to locate. An operation was deemed unnecessary.

As her symptoms gradually improved, her diet was extended and relaxed somewhat. Lucy was so convinced of the benefits of a macrobiotic lifestyle that she has continued to eat a macrobiotic diet, feels extremely well, has sorted out many emotional problems and feels very much in control of her life.

MARY

Mary, a thirty-four-year-old banker, said the reasons she made an appointment with a macrobiotic dietary counsellor were that she wished to rebalance her diet, which she had come to recognise as unhealthy. She was concerned for the future, because there was a family history of osteoporosis. Mary was low in iron and zinc; at the same time she was overweight and suffering PMS symptoms of moods, chocolate cravings and water retention .

A typical day's eating for Mary consisted of:

Breakfast Bread and butter and coffee
Mid-morning Coffee and a biscuit
Lunch Sandwich, crisps, yoghurt and coffee
Mid-afternoon Coffee, a chocolate biscuit (this was Mary's low energy period during the day)
Supper Pasta with creamy dressing, vegetarian sausages, frozen vegetables. A sugary pudding and coffee.

Mary regularly ate out late in the evening with friends, choosing similar food to that which she prepared at home— particularly pasta with oily, creamy toppings, and pizzas. When Mary arrived home hungry from work, she would go straight to the kitchen and start eating biscuits, bread and peanut butter, crisps and snacks. Her daily diet was high in fats, sugar, refined carbohydrates and empty calories—high-stress foods which had led to PMS symptoms and her being overweight. Her depression was suppressed with comforting foods, as well as alcohol and coffee. There was a lack of fresh, good quality, nourishing food.

Changing old eating habits and discouraging emotional dependence on food can be a difficult task. The changes for Mary were implemented very slowly, having regard to her absence from home during the day. She first discovered the qualities and goodness of vegetables and fruits. Stimulants were slowly reduced, her four to five daily cups of coffee being replaced by grain coffees and sugar by grain sweeteners. Good quality carbohydrates were also introduced, resulting in her feeling more energetic and less inclined to seek out a 'quick fix' in coffee and sugar, chocolate biscuits, etc.

Mary started to cook simple, nourishing meals with the help of cooking classes and regular advice from her counsellor, and learned to choose more nourishing, satisfying dishes in restaurants. Food eaten at lunch time was increased, so avoiding the need to binge on arriving home. Her new food included: wholemeal sandwiches with fillings of vegetarian pâté, smoked tofu or humous, tofu burgers, vegetable sticks, rice salad, hot soup in cold weather with some fresh fruit or seeds and dried fruit as a dessert.

Mary found that she could eat more, feel satisfied and at the same time was not putting on weight! (The fibre in the vegetables and fruit was having a cleansing effect.) Her life-long pattern of constipation was resolved in a few weeks as a result of eating more vegetables and wholegrains. If she was hungry during the day, she would eat vegetable slices or sticks, fruit, or sugarless biscuits and maybe drink a herbal tea. Reducing stimulants made her feel less stressed and more in control of her life. Mary's original problem of low minerals was balanced by first cutting down on all foods and drinks which deplete the minerals in the body—stimulants, sugar, chocolate and alcohol—then adding small amounts of good quality sea vegetables as part of daily meals. She got into the habit of eating supper at least two hours before going to bed, increasing her intake of good quality organic vegetables, such as greens, mushrooms, alfalfa sprouts, radishes, celery and root vegetables.

The changes needed to be complemented with some light exercise. Mary took up yoga and gentle walking at weekends; feeling more in tune with nature helped too. The PMS symptoms diminished slowly and finally disappeared. Her weight started decreasing at the same speed. Mary came to appreciate the benefits of eating supper much earlier and having a nourishing breakfast and lunch. One of the benefits she felt she had gained from her switch to a macrobiotic lifestyle was the conviction that it would prepare her, physically, mentally and emotionally, for her menopausal years ahead.

CHAPTER FOURTEEN

Reflexology

WHAT IS REFLEXOLOGY?

Reflexology is a hands-on therapy in which pressure and massage techniques are used to stimulate reflex points on the feet (and hands). The aim is to create a relaxed, dynamic healing effect in the body, to assist the release of blockages and maintain a balanced state of health at all levels.

The feet (and hands) are perceived as a mirror of the body, the left foot corresponding to the left side and the right foot to the right side. Placed together, the feet form a 'picture' of the body—from the area of the toes, which corresponds to the head and neck, down to the heel of the foot, which relates to the knees and the sciatic area. The anatomy of the body is understood to be divided into ten vertical and three horizontal energy zones. There is a direct link between these zones—and their associated organs and functions—and specific reflex points on the feet. Reflexology uses this link for therapeutic effect.

The principles and action of reflexology are similar to the system of qi (energy) and the meridian pathways of acupuncture/acupressure. There is also a close link between reflexology and Shiatsu (see chapter Eight).

Reflexology can help a wide variety of physical and emotional disorders, both acute and more deeply seated. Whilst it is a simple method of treating illness and maintaining good health, reflexology is also used to detect disharmony within the body and is therefore of great value in preventing ill health.

A BRIEF HISTORY OF REFLEXOLOGY

Therapeutic foot massage has been used all over the world for thousands of years. In Europe during the sixteenth century, medical practitioners made reference to the therapy. In the early part of the twentieth century, Dr William Fitzgerald, an American ear, nose and throat specialist, followed up the earlier references and laid the foundations for the development of modern-day reflexology. Dr Fitzgerald observed that pressure applied to specific areas of the feet and lower legs had an anaesthetising effect on certain parts of the body. He went on to develop this connection, establishing that the body could be divided into ten vertical zones, ending in the fingers and toes; linking the reflex areas on the feet (and hands) to the particular areas, organs and systems within each zone.

Dr Fitzgerald's work was further developed and refined by an American masseuse, Dr Eunice Ingham, who explored zone therapy as a means of treating the symptoms of ill health and relaxing the body in order to encourage self-healing. Her work did much towards establishing the modern method of reflexology.

More recently, during the 1960s a German therapist, Hannah Marquadi, determined that the body and feet could be further divided into three horizontal energy zones. Reflexology is now an extremely popular holistic method of healing and has joined others such as homoeopathy, spiritual healing and aromatherapy in mainstream health care.

TREATMENT

A reflexology session can be expected to last from twenty minutes to an hour. Treatment is received in a comfortable, reclining position. The practitioner normally concentrates on the feet—the soles, tops and sides—as the feet are more responsive to treatment than the hands.

Treatment begins with some relaxing warm-up techniques, followed by a set routine during which the practitioner uses the thumbs, fingers and hands to apply massage and firm pressure to the reflex points, paying extra attention to areas which indicate a blockage in the flow of energy. Blockages are determined by the patient's reaction to pressure (slight pain or tenderness may be felt), and the presence of very small areas of crystalline deposits just beneath the surface of the skin.

A typical course of reflexology treatment is six sessions. The practitioner does not diagnose, but may give guidance in order that specific reflexes can be worked on at home between treatments.

SELF-HELP FOOT AND HAND MASSAGE

Simple techniques that you can easily and safely carry out for yourself, or with a friend or partner, can help minor health conditions. If you wish to try reflexology for yourself, a quick, simplified massage routine to help relieve minor ailments, relax, tone and balance the whole body, is given below:

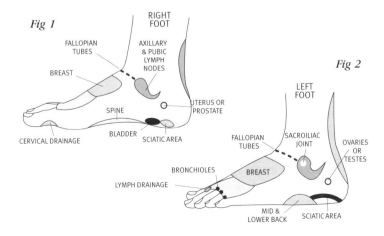

Fig 1

RIGHT FOOT

FALLOPIAN TUBES

AXILLARY & PUBIC LYMPH NODES

BREAST

Fig 2

UTERUS OR PROSTATE

SPINE

LEFT FOOT

BLADDER   SCIATIC AREA

CERVICAL DRAINAGE

FALLOPIAN TUBES

SACROILIAC JOINT

OVARIES OR TESTES

BRONCHIOLES   BREAST

LYMPH DRAINAGE

MID & LOWER BACK   SCIATIC AREA

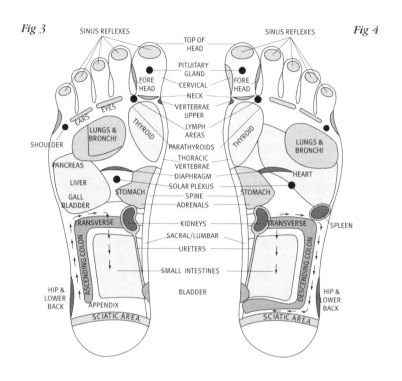

Fig 3   Fig 4

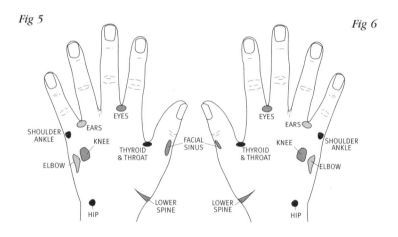

Fig 5   Fig 6

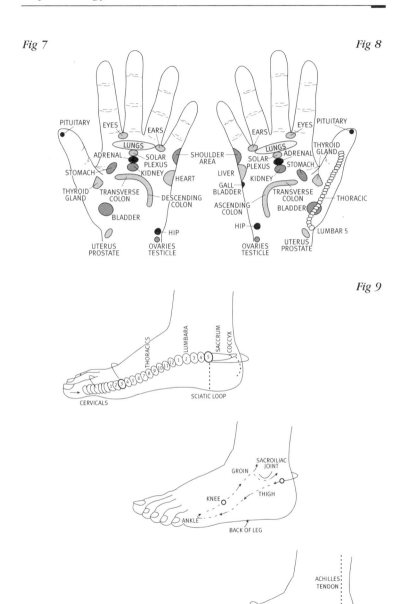

Fig 7

Fig 8

Fig 9

A Cautionary Note

Avoid having a heavy meal before treatment. Care should be taken when working on your own feet—bear in mind that over-stimulation could cause tension and imbalance. Do not persist with treatment if it feels *too* painful; this would indicate a blockage which should be investigated and treated by a trained reflexologist. Home massage should not be attempted if you suffer from varicose veins, phlebitis, kidney stones, thrombosis and heart problems. Avoid working on the kidneys and bladder if you have an acute incontinence problem; the uterus and ovaries if you have severe menstrual difficulties; the stomach if ulcers are present.

If a partner is working on your feet, you can recline, with the back well supported and the feet resting on a cushion, if you wish. If you are working alone, sit in a comfortable position—and relax. Rest the foot (or hand if it is easier), on the opposite thigh. If your feet look dry, rub in some moisturiser. Before commencing the routine, dust a little talc over the foot.

The feet (or hands) should be given a simple warm-up. Flex and extend the foot. Rotate it slowly for a few seconds, then rub the whole foot with the hands. In self-treatment it is easier to work with the top of the thumbs, using a circular motion. Work each reflex area for about five seconds, using a degree of pressure which would bruise a tomato. If tenderness is felt, release the pressure then return to the area, maintaining pressure for another five seconds until the pain diminishes. The blockage in the zone should then have cleared. During the routine, you may also detect very tiny lumps under the skin, which feel like crushed crystals. If worked on in a similar way to painful reflexes, it is likely they will disperse after one or two treatments.

Always start with the right food (or hand). Treatment should commence and finish with a few seconds' pressure to the solar plexus reflex. This is a tender spot on the sole of the foot and slight pain will be felt. Continue on the sole of the foot working on the thyroid area, which is at the base of the pad below the big toe (the base of the thumb on the hand). From the thyroid, starting with the big toe, massage the toes one by one. Drop down to the base of the toes for the eyes and the ears then across the pad for the lungs. Then work the liver, gall-bladder and stomach. Continue down the centre of the foot to the small intestine, following the arrow up the ascending colon and across the transverse colon. Move on to the adrenals, kidneys and ureter tube into the bladder. The spine is located on the inside of the foot (see illustrations). Hold the thumb on the position of lumber no. 5 then, with a linking action (see Fig. 9), stretch the middle finger over to the top of the other side of the foot. With a series of circular movements, keeping the thumb on lumber no. 5, work along the arrows, starting at the thigh and moving to the ankle, knee and groin. Move the thumb to thoracic no. 3, change the linking, working in the direction of the arrow on the shoulder elbow and wrist. Move on to the uterus, fallopian tube and ovary. Lastly, work the lymph glands on top of the foot, using the fingers to work with a dragging motion towards the ankle.

Working the left foot is the same as the right, but the liver and gall-bladder are missing. Instead, work the heart—gently. Remember to follow the direction of the arrows on the descending colon.

The reflex areas on the hands resemble those in the feet. If working on the hands, the same procedure should be followed.

SELF-HELP FOR SIMPLE MENOPAUSE SYMPTOMS
Ensure you run through the above routine before proceeding
with self-help for the symptoms set out below.

Breast Lumps Solar plexus, diaphragm, chest area, thoracic
(spine), lymph glands.
Constipation Solar plexus, small and large intestines
(ascending colon), adrenals, liver, gall-bladder, sciatic nerve.
Constipation responds well to reflexology, often with rapid
results.
Depression Solar plexus, head, brain, pituitary, thyroid,
adrenals, all toes.
Dizziness Solar plexus, diaphragm, all toes—especially
cervical and pituitary area, eyes and ears.
Dry Skin Thyroid and adrenals.
Eye Problems Eye reflexes under toes, throat/neck, liver,
kidneys, diaphragm.
Fatigue Adrenals, diaphragm, all glands, whole spine.
Fluid Retention Lymph system, kidneys, adrenals.
Headache Whole spine, diaphragm, all glands and toes
(rotate big toe), neck and cervical area, eyes.
Hot Flushes Thyroid, adrenals, pituitary, diaphragm,
reproductive system.
Haemorrhoids Diaphragm, all glands, rotate big toe.
Indigestion Solar plexus, thoracic (spine), stomach,
pancreas, liver, gall-bladder, intestines.
Menstrual Problems (irregularity, cramp, general)
Uterus, ovaries, fallopian tube, diaphragm, lower spine, all
glands, Achilles tendon.
Nervous Tension Solar plexus, whole spine, all glands,
diaphragm, adrenals.
Skin Problems (including acne and dry skin) Liver,
adrenals, diaphragm, kidneys, intestine, thyroid.

Urinary Problems (including incontinence and cystitis) Bladder/kidney/ureter, adrenals, lower spine, diaphragm.

Note For the more serious menopausal conditions, or those which do not respond to self-treatment, particularly where there may be underlying reasons for the problems, it is advisable to consult a trained reflexologist.

CASE HISTORIES

AMELIA

Amelia was in a low state of health when she asked a reflexologist for help. Six months previously, she had taken early retirement from teaching on the grounds of a deterioration in her mental health, but she still felt quite depressed. Her right shoulder was painful and she was also experiencing stomach pain after eating. This had caused her to adopt an erratic eating pattern. Amelia had always suffered from bouts of depression, especially following a viral infection, but she felt that her present condition, the problem with her digestion and possibly the pain in her shoulder could be connected to the menopause.

Whilst checking for contra-indications, the reflexologist noticed that Amelia's ankles were swollen, suggesting water retention. There were a few visible broken capillaries on the insteps of the feet. Looking at the body as a whole, the presence of spots and lesions indicated impurities under the skin. She was advised to increase her fluid intake immediately and drink plenty of pure water during the course of the day.

After the preliminary warm-up massage, a thumb walk through the zones and treatment of the solar plexus, the reflexologist noticed that the thyroid gland reflex area felt very granular, which she managed to disperse. Working on the shoulder reflex caused acute discomfort with pain shooting up Amelia's arm to the shoulder. Treatment was continued on this area until relief occurred.

Amelia indicated that she felt tenderness when the reflexes relating to the stomach, ascending colon and small intestine were worked. Similarly, with the kidney, ureter and bladder area, which tied in with her history of renal problems. When approaching the top of the foot, the lymph gland reflex felt painful and was given extra treatment to drain the excess fluids.

At her second treatment, Amelia reported that the pain in her right shoulder had eased slightly, allowing increased mobility and flexibility. She was now able to eat larger meals without experiencing any discomfort. Her delight and relief at the improvement in her symptoms had resulted in her feeling less depressed. Extra attention was given to the kidney, ureter and bladder areas and to the lymph gland area, as Amelia's ankles were still slightly swollen.

At the third consultation, Amelia reported that she had continued to drink more fluids; her skin had certainly improved—fewer spots and lesions being present. The swelling in her ankles had further reduced and walking was less painful. No pain had occurred after eating average-sized meals. On treating the feet, there was still discomfort in the reflex areas of the stomach, colon, small intestine, kidney, ureter and bladder. All areas indicating problems were given extra treatment.

Amelia appeared cheerful at the fourth consultation and said that she had been feeling much less depressed. She continues to see the reflexologist occasionally for a maintenance treatment.

PAMELA

Pamela had been through a very traumatic period over the previous two years, due to losing her husband from a heart attack and being left with problems over land and property which had to be resolved in a court of law. She had been married for twenty-eight years to a farmer. Her children had all left home, so she had moved to a smaller property. Unhappily, she had not settled there and was planning to move again.

At forty-eight, shortly after the death of her husband, Pamela developed physical and emotional symptoms. Her left wrist, elbow and shoulder felt painful on moving, especially when she was working outside in cold weather. She had also developed hot flushes and was suffering a high degree of perspiration, day and night. Emotionally, she felt out of balance and confused. Pamela had always enjoyed robust health apart from recurring kidney stones, and chose not to consult her GP on this occasion. Her daughter had benefited from reflexology, so she decided to ask a practitioner to visit her at home.

On examination of Pamela's feet for contra-indications, no significant signs were found apart from slightly abnormal perspiration levels. To begin, both feet were relaxed with a warming massage, followed by thumb walking zones 1–5 and the solar plexus until fully relaxed. It was observed that pain was experienced in the pineal, pituitary and thyroid glands, stomach reflexes and the kidney/ureter region. Special attention was paid to the latter, due to Pamela's problem with kidney stones. More treatment was also given to the big toes to assist with the confusion, and to the lymph reflexes on the sole and the top of the feet to help the perspiration. When working on the reflexes of the shoulder and arm Pamela experienced a sensation which she likened to pins and needles, beginning at the top of her left arm and extending down into her hand. At the end of this first treatment, pressure points were used to increase the release of energy into the area of the left arm. She also received advice on self-help hand reflexology for pain relief, which she carried out at home throughout the course of treatment.

At her second treatment, Pamela reported that she had been experiencing less pain and more flexibility in her arm. She was still feeling pain in the pineal and pituitary reflexes and a granular build-up was found in the thyroid region. The kidney and ureter area was still particularly painful and some pain was present in the area of the left shoulder, along with the 'pins and needles' sensation. Extra treatment was given to all these areas.

Pamela was thrilled to report at her third treatment that she had almost full mobility in her left arm and that she was able to put on her coat unaided. This had not been possible for the past six months. The intensity of the hot flushes and sweats had lessened and they were not occurring so frequently. Emotionally she felt more collected and less confused. Treatment was concentrated on the kidney/ureter, as Pamela was due to have an operation for the removal of kidney stones.

At the fourth and last session, Pamela reported that her arm had made a complete recovery, that the hot flushes were no longer a problem and that she felt much better in herself. Extra treatment was concentrated in the kidney/ureter area. Pamela said she felt that reflexology was a good way of relaxing, balancing and harmonising the body through the menopausal phase of life.

CHAPTER FIFTEEN

Relaxation

THE NEED TO RELAX

Most of us enjoy relaxing or taking a break, but many women experiencing menopause find it hard to admit they need to rest when tired and cannot adjust to slowing down, simplifying or making changes in their busy routines. Sadly, they fail to recognise and understand the detrimental effects of stressful symptoms on their health.

If you can see the benefits of leading a more relaxed life and implement changes to bring this about, you will be taking the first step to making your tension and unwanted worries disappear.

THE CAUSES, SIGNS AND EFFECTS OF STRESS

There are many influences which can bring about stress: bereavement, divorce, moving house, money problems, deep-seated emotional patterns, arguments, deadlines, incorrect diet, noise, travel, the weather, unsatisfactory situations. Sometimes it appears that there is little we can do about the onward march of our high-tech, computerised society with its pace-increasing hardware, such as mobile phones, facsimile machines, E-mail and the Internet.

The body acts as a teacher and is a barometer of your health. If you learn to listen to it, you can become more aware of how stress affects you. Take note of the simple signs— shoulders drawn up around the ears, clenched fists and jaw, headaches, aches and pains, insomnia, digestive disturbances, breath holding or rapid breathing, a faster pulse, panic attacks and all manner of minor ailments that can give rise to more serious symptoms such as high blood pressure, diabetes and other degenerative diseases. Important to the menopausal woman is the fact that not only does stress deplete the immune system, but it can cause hormonal imbalance—an unwanted complication at a time when your balance is already changing as part of a natural process.

It is true that you need a certain amount of tension in order to function properly. In fact, stress can have a beneficial and pleasant effect; improving confidence and ability when used positively to meet challenges and achieve goals. In preventing stress from becoming harmful, it is essential to be aware of the amount you can comfortably cope with and the point at which it could become a threat to your well-being.

Relaxation is one of many holistic approaches which can be used to help you look at and change negative patterns of behaviour which are causing stress in your life, and bring you to a point where you are in a better position to deal with problems. Those who are taking medically prescribed tranquillisers for stress and who wish to try other methods, should seek professional advice from their general practitioners first.

BENEFITING FROM RELAXING AND DEEP RELAXATION TECHNIQUES

To be in a relaxed state is a natural way of being, though most of us have lost the ability to regain a feeling of complete tranquillity for any length of time. Although many activities can provide short periods of respite and temporary freedom from tension, true relaxation brings the body to a point of complete calm, enabling it to re-balance and heal itself in whatever way is needed.

Consider some of the advantages and benefits which are possible.

Relaxing:

- when tired or at the first sign of illness, will prevent many stress-related ailments from developing
- facilitates clarity of mind, enabling you to work with greater efficiency and solve or put problems in order of priority
- provides inspiration and promotes creativity
- helps attain peace of mind, lifts depression, encourages restful sleep
- assists the body to revitalise and heal itself more quickly
- relieves tension, strengthens the system and brings relief to physical ailments, such as digestive upsets and headaches
- increases intuition and self-awareness—enabling unacceptable situations to be changed.

SUGGESTIONS AND GUIDANCE

Prolonged stress can lead to exhaustion and eventual breakdown of functions. Although it may feel frightening or challenging, take a long hard look at what is stressing you and, if necessary, seek help to bring about positive changes and make life easier.

In addressing the causes of stress, you may find it helpful to practise some form of relaxation every day. Consider whether you could be helped by these suggestions:

- if needed, take steps to develop confidence/assertiveness to enable you to say 'no'
- give attention to time management, and don't take on more than you can comfortably manage

- whenever possible, walk away from conflict
- replace negative thoughts and statements with positive ones. It is helpful to make this into an exercise on paper
- smile (this has a knock-on effect in the body) and act calmly
- get plenty of fresh air and sunshine, which is important for hormonal health
- take regular exercise, such as brisk walking (see Benefits of Regular Exercise below)
- consider joining a relaxation/exercise class or learning yoga or T'ai-chi (gentle Chinese slow motion exercises which aid posture)
- punch a pillow or dig the garden when angry
- aim for evenings to be a time of winding down. This will assist peaceful sleep
- share problems with someone willing to listen and don't be afraid to ask for help
- focus attention on one thing at a time
- visualise problems sorting themselves out as you would wish
- stop when tired, sit down, take a break or make a diversion
- make positive affirmations in the present tense:'I am now feeling healthy and full of energy'
- listen to relaxation, visualisation, self-awareness tapes— useful when the mind is too tired to do anything else
- if possible, take a holiday or change your routine
- listen to your body, be aware of posture, tension and faulty breathing. Ensure your sitting position is comfortable and relaxed (see Posture below)
- pamper yourself with a luxury—like a massage or a candlelit bath

- keep life as simple as possible, go with its natural flow and be ready to adapt to change
- eat a simple, healthy, wholefood diet in a relaxed environment. Avoid rushed meals. Ensure the food is chewed slowly and thoroughly. Don't overload the stomach. The lift obtained from coffee, alcohol, cigarettes, chocolate and sugary food has a damaging downside. Foods containing B complex vitamins help combat stress
- regularly make time to enjoy a hobby or leisure activity
- ensure you have adequate sleep. (Recent research has shown that the essential work of repair and cell renewal in the body is carried out during sleep.) If you have difficulty in falling asleep, the Total Body Relaxation routine, described below, might help.

BENEFITS OF REGULAR EXERCISE

Taking regular exercise and keeping the body fit can have far-reaching effects, helping to overcome problems, both physical and emotional. Regular exercise should form a lifelong habit for everyone, but it's never too late to begin. The benefits and rewards of appropriate exercise for the menopausal woman are manifold. Exercise:

- builds bone mass
- improves breathing action and functions of the lungs and heart, reducing the risk of heart disease, strokes and high blood pressure
- reduces the discomfort of hot flushes
- stimulates, tones and strengthens the whole system, lessening fatigue, improving suppleness, agility, balance and posture

- helps release and lessen anxiety and tension, creating feelings of well-being and positivity
- reduces depression
- promotes restful sleep
- relieves many physical problems, including constipation and menstrual cramps
- improves sex drive
- enables the body to deal with pain by activating endorphins—its natural painkillers
- helps to reduce weight
- helps the body to absorb calcium and other nutrients
- tones the digestive system. Reduces cravings for unhealthy foods
- increases suppleness and stamina
- improves skin tone and hair condition.

Regular exercise can be any activity practised at least four times a week, preferably daily, for at least half an hour. It should not exhaust you or put undue strain on any part of the body. Be aware that sporting exercise can be counter-productive and cause unwanted tension if the spirit of competition is taken to the extreme.

Some ideas include walking briskly, jogging, hill walking, swimming, dancing, cycling, keep fit, tennis/badminton, riding, golf and gardening.

POSTURE

Poor posture limits and strains the body, preventing it from functioning in the way it should. This can result in many health problems, such as tiredness, headaches, digestive disorders and pains in the neck, knees, shoulders and arms. We are born with the ability to hold ourselves well. Very young children display enviable posture. Sadly, most start to lose their poise around the time they start school.

One of the best methods of re-awakening the body and adopting good posture is yoga, which incorporates valuable breathing techniques. Another useful method is the postural training and poised movement of the Alexander technique. Both methods are successfully used in the treatment of many ailments.

New postural habits will probably feel strange at first, but your body will soon re-adjust. By aiming to achieve posture which is poised inside and out, not only can you achieve better health but you can reach a point of balance at which it will be possible for you to gain greater self-awareness.

Self-help Suggestions
Regularly monitor your posture, checking—in a mirror where possible—for tension, faulty positioning and slumping.

Stretching is a simple way of improving posture and relaxing tense muscles. It can be part of an exercise routine or done quickly, almost anywhere.

Stand upright with your back against a wall. Your body should feel comfortable and not be rigid. The back of your head, shoulder blades, buttocks and heels should all be touching the wall. Ensuring that your shoulders are down, your pelvis straight and feet pointing ahead, walk away in a relaxed manner. Keep practising until the habit comes naturally.

When sitting, ensure that the back of your chair is comfortable and will keep your back straight. Chair height should enable your feet to rest flat on the floor, pointing straight ahead. Keep your head in line with the back of the chair—avoid craning forward. Try not to let your head droop or fall to one side. Keep your chin level and your shoulders down. Don't hunch or twist them.

RELAXATION TECHNIQUES
There are many easily managed methods of relaxation, some very simple, others requiring more concentration. Choose from the following according to your ability and lifestyle.

QUICK EXERCISES FOR BUSY WOMEN
- Try stretching your whole body, then relaxing it. (Watch a cat's technique on rising!)
- Tense your whole body, then relax it (5 minutes)
- Breathe in and exhale, using a long sighing out-breath, three times (2 minutes)
- Bring your shoulders right up, then drop them, repeat three times
- Get into the habit of mentally scanning your body and releasing any points of tension. Increased safety can be one benefit. A nervous, tense driver is more likely to have an accident. Does sitting forward in a hunched position with hands clamped tightly on the steering wheel sound familiar?

SOME RELAXING YOGA EXERCISES

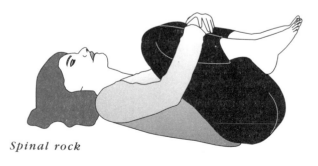

Spinal rock

1. Lie down on your back. Bring both your knees up together and clasp your hands behind or on top of them. Although very relaxing in itself, this can be a useful preliminary to the next exercise.

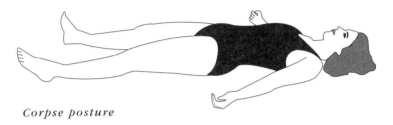

Corpse posture

2. The 'corpse' posture. Lie down on your back and close your eyes, ensuring that as much of your spine as possible is in contact with the floor. Your legs should be slightly apart, feet falling outwards and your arms a short distance from your body, palms upward. Relax your hands and allow your fingers to curl a little. Breathe deeply through your nose, releasing any tension. Imagine your whole body sinking into the floor. This posture is very revitalising, even if practised for five minutes or so.

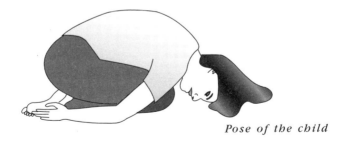

Pose of the child

3. The pose of the child. Kneel down and sit on your heels. Bend your body down slowly until your forehead touches

the floor. Bring your arms back, without stretching, and rest your hands (palms upward) on either side of your feet. Allow your shoulders to fall naturally and relax in this position.

4. Stand with feet slightly apart. Slowly lower your head, shoulders, arms and torso forward as far as is comfortable. Your arms should hang loosely; it's not necessary to touch your toes. Remain in this position for a few seconds, then unfurl slowly, making sure to straighten your head last. This exercise can even be done in the cloakroom at work!

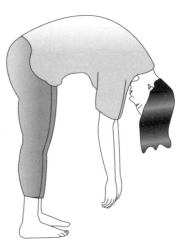

5. Consciously send your breath to the centre of your body (navel area), and hold the focus there. This is calming and will enable you to feel more in touch with yourself.

6. Standing or sitting, raise your shoulders and rotate them backwards ten to twenty-five times. Repeat, rotating the shoulders forwards.

7. Sit comfortably, close your eyes and lightly cover them with the palms of your hands for a few minutes. Focus on the blackness.

TOTAL BODY RELAXATION

Total body relaxation is intended to give the body and mind a complete rest. Practised regularly (daily if possible), an environment can be created for healing, allowing your true potential to be achieved. When using total body relaxation techniques, it is important to try to keep your mind clear of everyday thoughts and worries. However, should these occur, simply acknowledge them and let them go.

The place chosen for relaxation should be quiet, draught-free, comfortably warm, but not stuffy. You might choose to play some relaxing music. Clothing should be loose—there is no need to wear shoes. These techniques are normally done lying down. If using the floor, you can make yourself more comfortable by lying on a rug or folded blanket. A reasonably firm sofa or bed are also suitable.

A Total Body Relaxation Practice

Having made sure, as far as possible, that you will not be disturbed, lie down in the corpse posture (described above). Allow your eyes to gently close. Inhale deeply, then exhale with a long, slow breath. Relax. Remaining focused on your breathing, breathe normally for a few minutes. Observe the rise and fall of your abdomen and rib cage; the ebb and flow of the breath in your nostrils.

Take your attention to your right foot and tense it. Hold for a few seconds, then relax. Keeping the foot relaxed, tighten your whole leg—calf, knee and thigh. Hold, release and relax. Do the same with the left leg. Draw in the muscles of your buttocks, groin and pelvic floor. Pull in your abdomen, hold, release and relax. Move on to the chest and upper back. Tighten, release and relax. Move your attention to your right hand. Clench it into a fist, then release and keeping it relaxed, tighten your arm and shoulder. Release and relax. Repeat with your left hand, arm and shoulder. Tighten up the muscles of your neck. Hold, release and relax. Taking care not to overdo it, clench your jaw by holding your teeth firmly together, then purse your lips tightly. Close your eyes and frown as hard as you can. Feel the tension in the whole of your face and scalp. Hold, release and relax.

Be aware of how relaxed and peaceful you now feel. Remain lying down for as long as you wish, keeping your attention focused on your breathing. Gently bring your awareness back to the room and where you are lying. Open your eyes, have a good stretch and, when you are ready, slowly get up.

CASE HISTORIES

FIONA

Fiona was unhappy and stressed to the point where she wanted to scream. She had grown up in Liverpool and was one of seven children. Widowed in her early thirties with two young children, she had re-married at forty, to a naval officer, her third child being born when she was forty-one. Shortly afterwards, her husband was transferred to Portsmouth and the family moved south.

The new posting involved his being away from home for longer periods, which Fiona and the children found most unsettling. Fiona felt homesick for Liverpool and her family. She did not like Portsmouth and was finding it difficult to make friends. Most of her new neighbours were either out at work or retired.

At forty-seven, Fiona rarely felt she was on an even keel. Her two teenaged children had become insolent, uncooperative and selfish, rowing both with her and each other. Fiona found herself irritable for much of the time, frequently lashing out at the children during arguments. Pent-up feelings of resentment festered within her at being treated as an unpaid chauffeur and drudge in her own home.

Fiona wanted her husband's homecomings to be happy occasions and did her best to hide her distress from him. She loved him and was concerned that her desire to make love was decreasing. Fiona was deeply worried about this situation, and wondered if it was the beginning of the end of her sex life. She often comforted herself with chocolate and cake and also started to have a few glasses of wine before her evening meal to calm her nerves. Realising she was putting on weight and in an effort to feel more relaxed, she took up jogging. Although she had been keen on this in her twenties, she was dismayed to find how tired it now made her feel and gave it up.

Other problems mounted. These included hot flushes, headaches, bouts of crying and painful indigestion. Attributing many of Fiona's difficulties to her approaching menopause, her doctor suggested she relax more and offered tranquillisers. Fiona stopped taking these after a month as they did not suit her.

The turning point came when, after a little persuasion, she shared her problems with a visiting older sister, from whom she learned much more about the menopause and how her sister had dealt with problems. Fiona's first action after her sister left was to tell her husband what had been happening. After successful family counselling, problems with the children were resolved and home life became more harmonious.

Following her doctor's advice, Fiona looked at ways in which she could relax. She bought a bicycle, often using it in place of the car. She also took up T'ai-chi, setting aside a few minutes each day for practice. A new friend made at the T'ai-chi class recommended a nutritional therapist, whose prescription included dietary changes, herbal preparations and supplements. Fiona's sister lent her some relaxation and visualisation tapes and Fiona would often play one in the evening. She also bought some relaxing aromatherapy oils and added them to her bath. Lavender oil proved most useful for her headaches.

A year after starting her new relaxation and nutritional regimen, Fiona could honestly say that all her complaints, including the spare tyre round her waist, had gone. She had made new friends at the T'ai-chi class and felt more cheerful and optimistic. Her libido had returned and, apart from the occasional hot flush, she felt very fit and well.

JANET

Janet was dismayed on being told by her doctor that he thought she was having an early menopause. At forty-three, this seemed to be the last straw in a chain of painful events spanning a period of some fifteen years.

An unhappy marriage had ended in divorce five years earlier. Contact with her ex-husband had been severed and no maintenance received. Shortly after her divorce, Janet's parents had died, within a year of each other. Her relationship with them had been close and she was overwhelmed with shock and grief.

Janet was delighted when her new partner suggested they set up home together. They found a house to rent near the primary school attended by her two children and where she worked in the mornings as a classroom assistant. Her partner's divorce was made final, but with an order for heavy maintenance payments. This was a blow to them both. They did not know how they would manage in the future.

Janet's health went downhill from that point. Her periods became more painful and she started having hot flushes. Fear of the future and anxiety over their financial situation was causing her to shake whenever the problems were discussed. Janet felt tired most of the time. It was an effort to cook the evening meal.

Existing health problems precluded Janet from taking HRT. Her doctor prescribed Evening Primrose oil for her hot flushes. In addition, he arranged counselling which proved beneficial, enabling Janet to deal with her unresolved grief over the deaths of her parents and the fear stemming from the mental and physical cruelty she had experienced from her ex-husband.

Janet realised that she was not at all relaxed and asked her partner to give her regular massage. They went on to try some self-help aromatherapy, using oils to help with period pain and anxiety, and also set aside time for walking, swimming and reading. Dietary changes were implemented, with an increase in foods containing vitamins B and E.

Although Janet realised that there was no overnight solution to their financial problems, her attitude and health steadily improved to the point where she felt positive and able to cope with the situation.

WENDY

Wendy had been away from home nearly every other weekend for six months, visiting and helping look after her elderly parents who lived over a hundred miles away. Her husband remained at home looking after their two sons of thirteen and fifteen and the dogs. Wendy had a part-time job as a supermarket checkout operator. Her husband had worked for the last twenty-five years at a local shoe factory, but at fifty, the same age as Wendy, had been made redundant. This came as a great blow and made them very depressed. Their town had a high unemployment rate and the chances of his being able to find suitable employment locally were slim.

The weekends away from home were exhausting Wendy. Her menstrual cycle had been erratic for the last two years and, despite taking medication, she suffered recurring cystitis.

Wendy had a history of emotional problems and, since the news of her husband's redundancy, had been experiencing panic attacks with palpitations. Although a sizeable redundancy payment was expected, Wendy was extremely fearful, often irrational, about the future.

Knowing that a medical herbalist had helped a friend at the time of her menopause, Wendy consulted the same practitioner who successfully treated her cystitis. The herbalist also included medicine to help with Wendy's menstrual cycle and agitation, suggesting there was much Wendy could do to help herself through relaxation. Wendy bought a book on stress management, adopting many of the techniques suggested. On talking matters over with her parents, she was delighted and relieved when they decided it was time to sell their house and move into a warden-controlled flat near to her home.

Feeling more optimistic and positive, Wendy learned to swim. She also went to an over-fifties aerobics class once a week and, with her husband, joined a clog dancing group. His attitude calmed to the point where he decided to start a small business from a hobby and Wendy's parents offered financial help to get the scheme off the ground. Wendy has continued with her anti-stress programme. At fifty-two, she joined her husband in his new business and now feels energetic and confident.

CHAPTER SIXTEEN

Common Symptoms and Holistic Treatments

Menopause is viewed with dread by many women who fear they might suffer some of its more formidable reported symptoms. These form a long and varied list, although not all are attributable to the physiological process of menopause, but can be signs of the general ageing process or an imbalance of some kind.

It is not possible to predict how smooth your passage through menopause will be. However, there are certain circumstances and predisposing factors which are generally understood to have an influence on the severity of symptoms.

Helpful factors which may lead to a smoother transition include:
- periods started late
- no pregnancies or children
- unmarried or married late
- financially secure
- better education
- good nutrition and a balanced lifestyle.

Factors which can give rise to more severe symptoms being experienced include:
- history of pre-menstrual syndrome
- low body weight

- early menopause (this occurs following the removal of both ovaries e.g. in a full hysterectomy).

Other factors which can cause premature menopause include radiotherapy and chemotherapy treatment, sterilisation, severe trauma, excessive smoking, poor nutrition and some diseases such as multiple sclerosis and arthritis.

The temptation to turn straight to this chapter is understandable, but please bear in mind that there is much of value to be found elsewhere in the book. If you are tempted, and decide on a particular treatment for a specific symptom, then at least read the chapter relating to that therapy first. The most successful approach is to investigate the underlying causes *before* embarking on a course of action.

A POCKET CASE HISTORY: JOY

Joy's pocket case history is an example of a menopause symptom endeavouring to point out the presence of buried emotional stress. Her only disagreeable symptom was an unbearable burning sensation on the tongue.

When Joy's three children were all under five, she had been deserted by her husband for a women who was carrying his child. Joy left the matrimonial home with her children and was forced to live in reduced circumstances, with poor financial support thereafter. The other woman moved in with her husband, adopting an affluent lifestyle. The two families remained in the same village. Joy found the strength to get on with life, although deeply resenting what had happened and having to work so hard to support herself and the children.

Joy and her ex-husband went out of their way to avoid

each other for twenty years, until one of their daughters was about to marry. Joy held out the hand of friendship and forgiveness to her ex-husband and his second wife, inviting them to a pre-nuptial party, to which they came. The next day, Joy noticed that the problem with her tongue had improved dramatically. She was able to relate this change to her gesture and concluded that it had enabled her to release the pent-up shock, grief and prolonged resentment harboured for so long.

ABDOMINAL PROBLEMS

The two most likely causes of digestive disorders are nutritional imbalance and reaction to stress.

Self-help Measures

- Adopt a healthy, fibre-rich diet suited to nutritional requirements and work towards strengthening the intestinal tract. Those with poor digestion are better for having more hot food and drinks. Eat relaxed, unhurried meals at regular times. Taking a walk after a meal will aid digestion.
- Try aloe vera juice, which is helpful for all abdominal problems. Take one tablespoon night and morning. Following improvement, continue with a maintenance dose of one tablespoon daily.
- Avoid foods which disagree with you and those which encourage constipation, e.g. excess fat and dairy products, spicy foods, too much protein and salt. Also avoid wheat bran, as this is high in phytates which hinder absorption of certain minerals, including calcium. It is also irritating to the gut and can create other problems. Use linseed or oat bran instead.
- Try to get into a regular bowel routine, but avoid

laxatives. They won't solve the problem in the long term and could discourage natural bowel action. Constipation can also be a simple case of dehydration due to lack of water in the diet (see Good Food Guide on fluids). Drink plenty of plain water.

- Look at what might be stressing you and explore ways to make life more peaceful. Try some relaxation measures. Massage and shiatsu may help. There are specific curative yoga postures for constipation, haemorrhoids and digestive disorders. Walk more, or take other forms of exercise.
- Try herb teas—chamomile, peppermint or fennel if you experience bloating, flatulence and dyspepsia. Ginger tea can be helpful for digestive pain (this is also warming).
- Applying warm water compresses to the anal area will help relieve the pain of haemorrhoids. There is more likely to be a problem with haemorrhoids where there is a history of constipation. Improvement of digestive health is essential when endeavouring to rectify haemorrhoid problems.

Note If you are experiencing any abnormalities associated with bowel action or digestion, especially anal bleeding, you should seek medical advice.

Aromatherapy
Bloating and flatulence In 50ml almond oil, mix the following quantities of drops: Ginger (10), Peppermint (10), Sweet marjoram (15) and Lavender (15).

Gently massage the abdominal area at least twice daily, or as needed to relieve discomfort.

Dyspepsia In 50ml almond oil mix Peppermint (10),

Ginger (10), Sweet Marjoram (10), Lavender (12) and Roman Chamomile (8). Gently massage into the gastric area at least twice daily. If pre-mixed in a dropper bottle, 6–8 drops of these essential oils can be used for a warm compress; *or* make a warm compress using Peppermint (1), Ginger (1), Sweet Marjoram (2), Lavender (2) and Roman Chamomile (2).

Haemorrhoids After emptying the bowels or bladder, put 2 drops of Lavender, Geranium (1) and Cypress (1) in about 1 pint of tepid water in a basin or bidet and use fresh cotton wool to bathe the rectal area.

Blend for long-term use: in a 10ml dropper bottle mix Lavender (80) drops, Geranium (50), Cypress (50). Mix 4 drops in about 1 pint of tepid water and use as above.

Bach Remedies

Digestive disorders can arise as a result of emotions such as worry, irritability, fear and depression. Look at Agrimiony, Chicory, Heather, Red Chestnut, Vervain, White Chestnut if you think your digestive disorder relates to worry; Beech, Chicory, Holly, Vervain, Willow if you are concerned about irritability; Aspen, Cherry Plum, Mimulus, Red Chestnut, Rock Rose if you feel fearful, and also the remedies mentioned under despondency and despair in the section on depression in the Symptoms chapter. Remember to look at the whole picture of the personality and any trauma you might be holding in when choosing remedies. For instance feelings such as guilt, responsibility, homesickness, shock, lack of confidence might lie behind other emotional symptoms. The cause must also be treated.

Herbal remedies
Abdominal problems generally Dandelion root (*Taraxacum radix*), and Yellow dock (*Rumex crispus*).
Digestive tonic Cascara sagrada (*Rhamnus purshiana*)
Haemorrhoids Pilewort (*Ranunculus ficaria*).

Take a tepid, herbal sitz bath using strong yarrow or chamomile infusions. A large bowl or baby bath is ideal for home use. Immerse the bottom for 10–15 minutes. Use calendula ointment topically.

Homoeopathy
Bloating Lycopodium, China. Either remedy can be of use when the condition is worse after eating and better for movement.
Constipation The constitutional remedy is the best choice. Sepia can help, especially around the menopause.
Haemorrhoids usually respond to alternate doses of Nux vomica and Sulphur. Dosage: Take one 30c pill at night. Review and repeat if necessary.

Macrobiotic
Two of the major causes of abdominal problems are a diet high in refined foods and saturated fats and lack of chewing (see section on chewing). Return to simple eating patterns (see advice on diet). Eat one umeboshi plum (obtainable in health food stores) daily, mixed with grain. Drink chamomile, ginger, peppermint, fennel or thyme tea after meals.
Bloating For a while: use a very simple diet—grains, fish, lightly cooked vegetables and fruits. Reduce or avoid bread and flour products, fruits and salads, curry, spices, sugar, refined carbohydrates, potatoes, beans and nuts and wheat products.

Constipation Increase whole, unrefined foods and all varieties of vegetables; those which are especially high in fibre are spring greens, kale, broccoli, watercress, green cabbage. Have some stir-fried vegetables daily, adding a little grated fresh ginger towards the end of cooking. Use ginger often in cooking. Make jellies using agar-agar. Use umeboshi plums, paste or vinegar in cooking.

Haemorrhoids Change from eating modern snacks and junk foods to unrefined wholefoods.

BODY TEMPERATURE CONDITIONS/ CIRCULATORY PROBLEMS

HOT FLUSHES/NIGHT SWEATS

Experienced in varying degrees of intensity and frequency by the greater proportion of menopausal women, hot flushes and night sweats can last from a few seconds to periods of up to an hour. They can occur over a period of months or years—sometimes extending into a woman's sixties and even beyond. Some women also experience accompanying anxiety, panic attacks or palpitations. Hot flushes are certainly the most discussed and best-known of all menopausal symptoms. The condition is understood to occur as a result of fluctuating hormone levels.

The liver has the task of ensuring the free circulation of blood throughout the body. Problems with body temperature and circulation are more likely to arise when there is an imbalance in liver function.

Much can be done holistically to alleviate the unpleasant symptoms of hot flushes and night sweats, from the simple measures of keeping cool and eating cooling foods, drinking plenty of plain water, relaxation and meditation techniques to specific therapeutic treatment.

Aggravating factors include: stress, hot weather, caffeine, alcohol, smoking, very hot drinks, spicy food, drugs and sugar. Regular exercise will help reduce symptoms. Stress reduction techniques are of value (see Chapter Fifteen Relaxation). Healing will also aid relaxation.

Aromatherapy
Make an aromatic bath: Add the following quantities of drops to a bath: Geranium (2), Lavender (3), Cypress (2), Clary sage (2) and Peppermint (1).

Body oil blend: 30 drops in 50ml of sweet almond oil: Roman Chamomile (5), Rose Maroc (10), Geranium (10) and Clary sage (5).

Blend of drops for long-term use: in a 10ml dropper bottle mix Geranium (35) Lavender (55) Cypress (35) Clary sage (35) and Peppermint (10). Add 6 drops to a bath.

Bach Remedies
Consider the following remedies when hot flushes stem from anxiety and tension or cause personal embarrassment:

- Agrimony: type has cheerful disposition, hides inner anxiety
- Impatiens: type is irritable, impatient and nervous
- Mimulus: type is fearful of known things, nervous, shy, blushes easily, likely to hide anxiety
- Larch: type is self-conscious and lacking in confidence.

All the physical symptoms listed under Body Temperature Conditions/Circulatory Problems may be helped by the Bach Flower Remedies which, in addition to being taken internally, can also be added to water and applied externally as a lotion.

Follow the advice given in Selecting Remedies for the Menopause in the Bach Flower Remedies chapter.

Herbal remedies
Body temperature conditions generally: Red sage (*Salvia officinalis*), Motherwort (*Leonurus Cardiaca*), Valerian (*Valeriana officinalis*), Chasteberry (*Vitex agnus castus*), Ladies Mantle, (*Alchemilla vulgaris*) (itchy skin), Dandelion herbal juice (night sweats).

Homoeopathy
The constitutional remedy is the best choice, but the following may be considered. (Dosage: 1 30c pill taken at night. Review and repeat if necessary.)
Lachesis: Flushes start when menstruation ceases, affecting face, head and neck area. Inclined to be sad and irritable, worse after sleep, from heat and pressure of clothing. Hot perspiration.
Sepia: Flushes start from the pelvic region. With perspiration and weakness. Depression, nausea, loss of appetite. Worse morning and evening.
Sulphur: Profuse perspiration all over. Hot in bed—night sweats.
Sumbul: With palpitations, worse from active exercise.

Natural Progesterone
This may be of help. Seek practitioner advice first.

Nutrition
A diet that is cooling will often help.
Reduce or cut out hot spices (pepper, chilli, curry, mustard), salt and highly salted foods (use low-salt products obtainable

from health food shops), tomatoes, sour foods (sour fruits, vinegars and vinegary foods such as pickles, yoghurt, etc.) oily or fatty foods, red meat, smoked or salted fish, shellfish, caffeine drinks (tea, coffee, cola) sugar, chocolate, cocoa, nuts (seeds are a good alternative) and alcohol.

Eat more a variety of fresh vegetables and fruits, rice and whole grains, coriander (fresh and dried), saffron, turmeric, fennel, rose water, peppermint and sage (in moderation—in tea or cooking), pulses, white meat (organic chicken and turkey), fresh fish, low-fat dairy produce, a little coconut, aloe vera juice—one teaspoon before meals and at bedtime. If there is a GLA deficiency, Evening Primrose oil can bring relief. Supplements include B complex, plus extra B5, magnesium and calcium.

DIZZINESS
Dizziness can occur as a reaction to stressful circumstances. It can also relate to hypoglycaemia or to postural hypotension (low blood pressure aggravated by movement). Being rendered 'off balance' might also be a body/mind message—a reminder that your life is out of balance in some way. If dizziness is persistent, is associated with the hearing or is giving rise for concern, seek medical advice.

Self-help Measures
- Endeavour to raise your general level of fitness
- Aim to reduce stress in your life—try relaxation and breathing techniques
- Try having a glass of water and mentally grounding yourself (see Meditation chapter)
- T'ai-chi or specific curative yoga exercises can be very beneficial to people prone to dizziness

Aromatherapy

Add to a bath: Lavender (2) and Peppermint (2).

Massage 2 drops of neat Lavender into the temples— avoiding the eyes—and around the front and back of the ears.

Blend for long-term use: In a 10ml dropper bottle mix Lavender (120) and Peppermint (60). Add 6 drops to a bath.

ITCHY SKIN
Aromatherapy

Add to a bath Blue (German) Chamomile (2) and Lavender (4). Add Blue Chamomile (4) and Lavender (6) to 50ml of unperfumed lotion to smooth into the skin when needed.

Blend for long-term use: in a 10ml dropper bottle mix Blue Chamomile (60) and Lavender (120) and add 6 drops to a bath. Also mix 10 drops of this blend in 50ml of unperfumed lotion to smooth into the skin when needed.

Nutrition

There may be a B vitamin deficiency or allergy. Itchy skin could possibly relate to the nervous system and stress. (See references to nervous system.)

BURNING MOUTH
Aromatherapy

Blend for long-term use: in a 10ml dropper bottle mix tincture of Myrrh (120), Peppermint (20), Lemon (30) and Eucalyptus (10). Mix 3 drops in a small cup of warm water and rinse mouth well.

Note Must not be swallowed.

For short-term use: add 1 drop of each of the above oils to a small cup of warm water.

Nutrition

Burning mouth or feet relate specifically to B vitamin deficiency.

PALPITATIONS

The feeling that the heart is beating much faster than it should can be very frightening. However, this is not normally a sign of a serious medical problem. Palpitations often accompany hot flushes and night sweats, can occur after strenuous exercise and have a well-known link with stress and digestive disorders.

General Self-help

These measures should include looking into the cause of the reaction, and techniques for stress relief.

Note It does not follow that there is a problem with heart disease if you experience palpitations, but if symptoms are severe and are accompanied by breathlessness, pain and dizziness, you should consult a medical practitioner.

Aromatherapy

Inhale Neroli (2) and Lavender (2) from a tissue. Vaporise Ylang Ylang (2), Lavender (2) and Petitgrain (2) in a burner or diffuser. Add the following quantities of drops to a bath: Lavender (2), Petitgrain (2), Ylang Ylang (1), Neroli (1). Make a body oil with Lavender (8), Petitgrain (8), Ylang Ylang (6) and Neroli (6) in 50ml of almond oil. Blend for long-term use: in a 10ml dropper bottle mix Lavender (50), Petitgrain (50), Ylang Ylang (40), Neroli (40) and add 6 drops to a bath.

Bach Remedies

Consider the type remedy and appropriate tension/anxiety

remedy (see Bach Remedies advice given under Hot Flushes). There is usually an element of fear involved, in which case choose from the following:

- Aspen Shows fears of unknown origin—no real basis. Anxious, apprehensive
- Mimulus Has known fears. Type is normally shy and retiring
- Red Chestnut Anxious about the welfare of others
- Rock Rose Has feelings of terror (known reason). Remedy of emergency.

Herbal Remedies
For circulatory problems generally Cramp Bark (*Viburnum Opulus*), Hawthorn Berry (*Crataegus Oxyacanthoides*), Prickly Ash (*Zanthoxylum*)

Homoeopathy
Aconite: Where there is fear present, or Ignatia if emotionally distressed. Nux vomica when there is a digestive upset. Dosage: 1 30c pill. Review and repeat if necessary.

Nutrition
Palpitations can be due to magnesium and/or calcium deficiency (see nutritional recommendations for supplementation under Osteoporosis). They can also relate to deficiency of B vitamins and vitamin C with bioflavenoids. People with heart problems and who are taking heart or blood pressure medication should consult a practitioner before using supplements.

LEG CRAMPS
Leg cramps may occur as a result of poor circulation or an

underlying circulatory disorder, in which case practitioner help should be sought. See also self-help measures to improve circulation suggested in section on varicose veins, and measures to calm the system generally and before bedtime (see sections on fatigue and insomnia).

Aromatherapy

Add the following quantities of drops to a bath: Lavender (3), Sweet Marjoram (2) and Roman Chamomile (2). Also massage feet, legs, hips and buttocks with a body oil—Lavender (1), Rosemary (8), White Thyme (6) and Roman Chamomile (6) in 50ml of sweet almond oil.

Blend for long-term use: in a 10ml dropper bottle mix Lavender (75), Sweet Marjoram (50) and Roman Chamomile (50) and add 8 drops to a bath.

Bach Remedies

• Impatiens: Pain caused by tension.

Herbal Remedies

Drink chamomile, ginger, thyme, sage or rosemary teas, take 1 teaspoon valerian tincture every two hours. Gently massage the area—wring out small towels in hot and cold water and apply alternately.

Homoeopathy

Cuprum met.: Dosage: Take 1 30c pill at night. Review and repeat if necessary.

Macrobiotics

Reduce liquid intake, raw salt on food or in salty snacks.

Nutrition

There may be a vitamin B6 deficiency which could be due to magnesium and/or calcium deficiency (see recommendations for supplementation under Osteoporosis). Hypoglycaemia and low thyroid activity or osteoporosis might be involved, and it is worth being checked. Try magnesium supplementation first, as this may solve the problem.

VARICOSE VEINS AND ULCERS

Some women are troubled during the change of life by varicose veins; ulcers might also develop. Varicose veins are normally associated with the legs, but they can occur in other parts of the body. Preventative and simple self-help measures to improve diet, the elasticity of vein walls and muscle tone may be considered:

- wear comfortable shoes and avoid standing for long periods
- lie down with the feet elevated above chest level for a few minutes each day
- bathe the area with cold water
- avoid being overweight
- exercise more—take plenty of brisk walks
- ensure that your diet is wholesome
- introduce more fibre-rich foods (e.g. fresh vegetables) to prevent constipation
- try specific yoga exercises for this condition and circulation generally. However, if you suffer from high blood pressure avoid inverted postures
- have a massage
- if there is accompanying itching, try Bach Flower Remedies Rescue Cream or calendula cream

- apply neat Witch Hazel to the affected areas
- avoid sitting with the legs crossed
- when sitting with the feet flat on the floor, raise the heels from time to time.

Aromatherapy

Add the following quantities of drops to a bath: Lemon (1), Lavender (3) and Geranium (3). Make an oil to be smoothed gently into the legs and ankles and more vigorously into the abdomen, hips and buttocks, with Lavender (12), Cypress (6), Lemon (6) and Geranium (6) in 50ml of sweet almond oil.

Blend for long-term use: in a 10ml dropper bottle mix Lemon (25), Lavender (75) and Geranium (75) and add 6 drops to a bath.

To help heal ulcers, very gently apply Lavender (3) in one teaspoon of Bach Flower Remedies Rescue cream.

Homoeopathy

Pulsatilla, Carbo veg. or Hamamelis: Also available as a cream. Dosage: 1 30c pill. Review and repeat if necessary.

Nutrition

Use vitamin C with a high level of bioflavenoids, vitamin E and gingko biloba. Also work on nutrition for weak connective tissues (see under Genito-urinary) and circulation.

Poor circulation Might relate to a deficiency of GLA. Vitamin C with a high level of bioflavenoids may help. Also, linseed or fish oil, lecithin, CoQ10, gingko biloba and a low dose (100iu) of vitamin E.

BONE PROBLEMS
STIFFNESS IN JOINTS, GENERAL ACHES AND PAINS

Around the menopause, some women notice they are more affected by aches and pains in the muscles and joints. The joints which score high in this respect are the elbows, knees and shoulders. Joint pains can arise from a host of causes—some short-lived, others more deep-seated and serious, such as arthritis or osteoporosis.

With the right care beforehand, bone problems during menopause can be prevented. Primarily, preventative action should focus on raising the general level of health, taking plenty of regular exercise, ensuring there is adequate absorption of calcium and magnesium and encouraging the healthy functioning of the parathyroid gland.

If you are already experiencing bone problems, some pointers might help to unravel more simple causes. First look at dietary and lifestyle factors:

* is your diet healthy and balanced?
* is your lifestyle positive and fulfilling?
* are you eating foods (or drinking alcohol) which can create a build-up of acid in the joints? Well-known culprits are tomatoes, citrus fruits and juices, sugar, coffee, dairy products
* are there too many salty foods in your diet?
* are you obtaining sufficient exercise?
* is the stiffness of body perhaps coming from a tension, or rigidity of mind?

Aromatherapy
General treatment for all symptoms of bone problems: Add the following quantities of drops to a bath: Lavender (2),

Juniper berry (2), Benzoin (2), Roman Chamomile (2) and Ginger (1).

Body oil blend: Lavender (10), Juniper berry (7), Benzoin (5), Roman Chamomile (5), Ginger (3) to 50ml almond oil.

Blend for long-term use: in a 10ml dropper bottle mix Lavender (55), Juniper berry (40), Benzoin (3), Roman Chamomile (30) and Ginger (25). Add 6–8 drops to a bath. Also make a body oil with 30 drops of this blend to 50ml of almond oil. For smaller areas such as the knees, lower back or wrists only, make a stronger oil with 50 drops in 50ml of almond oil.

Bach Remedies

* Rock Water: rigid mindedness, self-repression and denial, for tightened-up person with high standards.

Herbal Remedies

Celery (*apium graveolens*), helps discharge accumulated waste which can lead to stiffness

Prickly Ash (*Zanthoxylum*), stimulates circulation—very relevant to stiffness

Mexican Wild Yam (*Dioscorea villosa*), anti-inflammatory.

Homoeopathy

Stiff, painful joints and general aches:

Rhus tox

Worse: for rest, cold, at night, in damp weather, on first beginning to move.

Better: for warmth, and gentle, slow motion

Ledum

Worse: at night, heat of the bed.

Better: for cold applications.

Osteoarthritis of small joints of hands:
Calc. fluor.

Pains around the shoulders worse when actually bleeding:
Cimicifuga

Muscular aching:
Arnica
Worse: from touch, motion, damp, cold.
Better: lying down or with the head low.
Dosage: 1 30c pill taken at night. Review and repeat if necessary.

Nutrition
Stiffness in joints, aches and pains:
If there is no improvement after treatment for calcium and magnesium deficiency, consider the possibility of food sensitivity (allergy). GLA and linseed (flax seed) oil as a supplement may also be necessary. Hypoglycaemia can cause joint aches and pains. Aloe vera can help certain types of joint pain. Try taking 1 tablespoon daily.

OSTEOPOROSIS
The mineralised connective tissue which makes up the skeleton of the body is constantly being renewed. There are two types of bone cells responsible for this process—osteoclasts, which detect and dissolve older bone, and osteoblasts, which make the new bone, filling the space left for it. For bone to remain healthy, the osteoclasts and osteoblasts must remain in balance.

Lack of progesterone prevents the osteoblasts from making new bone; gradually, the bone becomes increasingly porous at a time of life when it is naturally losing porosity. The resulting disease, osteoporosis, does not manifest in the majority of cases until between the ages of fifty-five to sixty, but it has been developing surreptitiously for the previous twenty to thirty years as a result of incorrect/poor diet and lifestyle, lack of proper exercise and deficient hormonal health. Most women are unaware they have the disease until there is a significant break, or they discover a loss of height.

Risk factors include
- women of Caucasian descent
- slim women and those with a history of anorexia nervosa
- early menopause
- women who have not had children
- lack of exercise
- the use of steroids and other drugs
- markedly underweight or overweight
- family history of osteoporosis
- heavy smoking and alcohol drinking
- high protein, high sodium diet
- an excess of dietary fat (especially from animal sources) processed food, sugar and other acid-forming foods (including dairy), carbonated drinks, caffeine
- diabetes
- inadequate calcium intake. Many things can adversely affect the absorption of calcium in the body, including dairy products, sugar, honey, jams, etc., animal protein, foods from the nightshade family, carbonated drinks, alcohol and coffee, citrus fruits, vinegar, salt, stress.

Natural methods have proved very successful in the prevention, treatment and even reversal of osteoporosis. The foundations of good bone health are laid during the early years. Below are some of the influences which affect the growth of strong bones:

1. A diet which allows calcium, other minerals and trace elements to be absorbed. Calcium neutralises acid in the stomach; if excess acid is produced, calcium could be leached from the bones to neutralise it. Proper functioning of the endocrine glands, especially the parathyroid, which balances the metabolism of minerals. The parathyroid benefits from plenty of fresh fruit and salads.
2. Good blood circulation, which depends on sufficient exercise.
3. Sunshine. This works with calcium to create healthy bones.
4. It is possible that osteoporosis is less common or severe in those on a meat-free diet. Unless meat is organically produced, it might contain hormones which could have a negative affect on human hormones.

Homoeopathy
Aching due to thinning of the bones:
Calc. fluor.
Dosage: One 30c pill taken at night. Review and repeat if necessary.

Natural Progesterone
See Chapter Four Natural Progesterone. Seek practitioner advice first.

Nutrition

Use supplements of magnesium and vitamin D as well as calcium with boron.

BREAST SORENESS

Fullness and soreness of the breasts normally occur as a response to fluctuating hormone levels. Most women are affected pre-menstrually or during pregnancy. The discomfort can also be experienced during the change of life.

Another common breast problem, but nevertheless quite frightening, is the formation of small, benign breast lumps which are more painful pre-menstrually. This condition affects only a small percentage of women. It is more likely to occur in the mid-thirties or forties and usually disappears when menopause has passed. The vast majority of breast lumps are not malignant.

Holistic treatment of breast problems takes into account many factors, but the main areas for exploration are hormonal health, diet/nutrition and water retention, which has a relationship to hormonal balance. A practitioner is best placed to deal with problems relating to excess oestrogen or lack of progesterone and other hormonal imbalances. Self-help is best directed to improving the diet (see also self-help advice in Water Retention section), and having plenty of exercise, which will promote lymph drainage.

In the case of breast lumps, congestion is possibly made worse by the use of under-arm antiperspirants (that prevent you sweating) and by lymphatic congestion generally in this area. Use natural deodorants obtainable from health food shops, e.g. natural mineral deodorant stones. Use skin brushing and massage (lymph drainage). Vitamin C also helps, as does a clean diet and bowel.

Aromatherapy

Add to the bath Geranium (2) and Lavender (4). Make cool compresses with Roman Chamomile (1), Geranium (2) Cypress (1) and Lavender (2). Mix the same quantities in 2 teaspoons of sweet almond oil to gently smooth into the breasts and underarms.

Herbal Remedies

Chasteberry (*Vitex agnus castus*) is the main remedy, possibly used with a diuretic, i.e. Dandelion leaf or a lymphatic agent, e.g. Cleavers (*Galium aparine*).

Homoeopathy

Evening Primrose or Starflower oil are recommended.

Also, homoeopathic Phytolacca: breasts are painful and swollen, feel hard and lumpy, particularly before or during menstruation.

Worse: in wet, damp, cold weather; for movement.

Better: for warmth, rest and in dry weather.

Dosage: 1 30c pill taken at night. Review and repeat if necessary.

Nutrition

Can be helped with GLA, vitamin E. Avoid using hydrogenated margarines and cooking oils. Olive oil or unheated polyunsaturated oils are acceptable.

EYE PROBLEMS

Eyes act as a mirror of ourselves, reflecting back or manifesting problems which are occurring inside the body. In Traditional Chinese Medicine, the eyes are considered to be related to the liver, which regulates the blood supply. When the liver is not functioning as it should, various physical and emotional problems may develop, including eye disorders. Kidney disharmony may also contribute to eye problems. Professional practitioners are best placed to help with these imbalances.

Dry or sore eyes might occur in later life as a result of the natural decrease in body fluids (see Skin and Hair Changes for further information and help).

Herbal Remedies
Bathe the eyes once or twice a day with a solution of 1 drop of calendula tincture to a small wine glass of boiled lukewarm water.

Homoeopathy
Bathe the eyes once or twice a day in a solution of Euphrasia (eyebright) tincture. Add 1 drop of tincture to a small wine glass of boiled lukewarm water. Euphrasia is also available in tablet form. Take 6c or 30c. (6c can be repeated more frequently than 30c.)

Nutrition
Many eye problems are related to poor circulation from and to the eyes, which can become worse as you get older, due to arteriosclerosis. In this instance, nutrition to help arteriosclerosis and circulation generally would be helpful— see section on circulation. In particular, CoQ10, lecithin, rutin and vitamin C, with high levels of bioflavenoids, help circulation. If you also have high blood pressure, consult a nutritional therapist.

Dry or sore eyes Try supplementing with vitamin B complex, vitamin E, GLA, vitamin A.

FATIGUE, INCLUDING INSOMNIA AND DISTURBED SLEEP

When examining causes and ways of combating physical and mental fatigue, first take a look at how well you are coping with stress. Short-term, prolonged or suppressed stress can often lie behind health problems such as depression, adrenal and kidney depletion and low blood sugar—to all possible causes of fatigue.

Anaemia is commonly associated with fatigue; other causes include faulty digestion and Seasonal Affective Disorder (SAD). A factor which can easily be overlooked is the ever-increasing number of pollutants present in food and the environment.

Self-help Measures
* Eat a nutritious wholefood diet, having regard to the seasons and the energetic value of food. This will go a long way to providing quality fuel for the body
* Avoid becoming constipated
* Take a break or rest if you feel tired
* Use relaxation and meditation techniques
* Try the specific curative yoga postures for fatigue
* Alleviate lethargy or boredom by taking up a discipline or creative hobby
* During the daytime, have plenty of fresh air, sunlight and exercise
* In colder weather, keep warm, get more sleep, conserve energy and take things more easily.

Note If, despite taking measures to address fatigue, it still continues, seek practitioner help; unresolved emotional issues or a more serious underlying physical reason may be involved, such as anaemia, thyroid imbalance, diabetes or M.E.

Aromatherapy
Make an aromatic bath with the following quantities of drops: Geranium (2), Pine needle (2) and Bergamot (2).

Body oil blend: Geranium (10), Pine needle (8) and Bergamot (7), in 50ml of almond oil.

Blend for long-term use: in a 10ml dropper bottle mix the following quantities of drops: Geranium (50), Pine needle (60) and Bergamot (60). Add 6–8 drops to a bath and also make a body oil with 30 drops of the blend in 50ml of almond oil.

Bach Remedies
- Centaury: Subservient type, finds it difficult to say no and accordingly overtaxes strength. Becomes easily tired and drained of vitality.
- Clematis: Dreamy, indifferent type, preoccupied with own thoughts. Listless, needs a lot of sleep.
- Elm: Normally capable and confident. Can become exhausted through effort. Feels overwhelmed by responsibility and subsequently doubts ability to manage. Symptoms are temporary.
- Hornbeam: Tiredness of mind. 'Monday morning' feeling. Uncertain of capability to overcome problem, but usually succeeds in doing so.
- Oak: Resilient, courageous, dependable type. Hides tiredness or ill-health, struggles on regardless of body's need for rest.
- Olive: Complete exhaustion of mind and body, following prolonged hardship or illness.

- Sweet Chestnut: Exhaustion with extreme feelings of hopelessness and despair.
- Vervain: Highly strung type. Enthusiastic, active mind. Overworks and loses strength.
- White Chestnut: Cannot switch off worrying thoughts going round and round in the mind, which can cause sleeplessness, exhaustion and depression.
- Wild Rose: Resigned to ill-health, apathetic. Always tired— gives up easily.

Homoeopathy
The constitutional remedy is best advised. Physical fatigue can respond to Phosphoric acid. Dosage: Take 1 30c pill at night. Review and repeat if necessary.

Nutrition
Fatigue can be due to candida overgrowth or food sensitivity (allergy). Adrenal depletion and hypoglycaemia—low blood sugar are also possible causes, as is deficiency of certain vitamins, minerals or other nutrients. B complex and magnesium, along with GLA (the active ingredient of Evening Primrose oil), CoQ10 (Co enzyme Q10) can all be very helpful in fatigue. It is also useful to have a blood test for anaemia if fatigue persists.

INSOMNIA AND DISTURBED SLEEP
Insomnia and disturbed sleeping patterns are problems which affect everyone at some time. Causes are numerous and often difficult to pinpoint for the individual. For those who are prone to sleep disorders, the menopause can bring yet more problems likely to influence sleeping—hot flushes, night sweats, indigestion, aches and pains, haemorrhoids,

panic attacks and depression.

Resorting to sleeping pills, which have the disadvantage of possible side-effects, even addiction, will not cure or get to the bottom of the problem. Taking first place in the list of causes must be worry and tension. Self-help de-stressing measures could include sharing your problems with a counsellor, gradually winding down activities during the evening, keeping to a simple, relaxed routine, using a relaxation/meditation/creative visualisation technique or enjoying a massage. Try some herbal sedative tablets or teas, such as valerian, chamomile or elderflower, obtainable in health food shops.

Avoid stimulating the system late in the evening with, for instance, late evening discussion and television viewing, hot baths, stimulating aromatherapy treatment after 7.00 pm or active exercise. It is more beneficial to exercise during the day. It is also better to avoid eating large meals late in the evening or drinking too much of any fluid, but especially alcohol, tea, coffee, colas, cocoa, etc. (stimulating drinks contribute to tension, hot flushes and body temperature conditions).

Aromatherapy

Add the following quantities of drops to a bath: Lavender (3), Clary Sage (2) and Ylang ylang (2). Avoid using alcohol when using Clary sage, as it can produce over-vivid dreams. After a bath, also massage 1 drop of Vetivert into the chest and solar plexus with a gentle anti-clockwise motion.

Blend for long-term use: in a 10ml dropper bottle mix Lavender (75), Clary sage (5), Ylang ylang (50) and add 6–8 drops to a bath.

Bach Remedies

- Agrimony: Hides worries behind a brave face. Mental anguish. Restless in bed. Churning thoughts causing insomnia.
- Aspen: Anxiety, apprehension and fear, by day or night, with no logical explanation.
- Honeysuckle: Inclined to live in the past. Regrets. Pessimistic about present and future. Difficulty sleeping due to grief (useful bereavement remedy combined with Star of Bethlehem).
- Impatiens: Impatient—irritated by slowness. Sleeplessness caused by tension and restlessness.
- Mimulus: Fear (of known things) prevents restful sleep. Shy, retiring type. Inclined to hide anxiety and fear.
- Olive: For complete exhaustion of mind and body, following prolonged hardship or illness. Cannot sleep for overtiredness.
- Rock Rose: Difficulty in sleeping owing to feelings of panic, extreme fear (known reason).
- Rock Water: Sleeplessness through tension. Rigidity of outlook. Self-repression—denial.
- Star of Bethlehem: Sleeplessness through grief, sorrow, grievous disappointment, shock.
- Vervain: Highly strung type. Enthusiastic, active mind. Restless in bed.
- White Chestnut: Cannot switch off from worrying thoughts going round and round in the mind, which can cause sleeplessness, exhaustion and depression.

Herbal Remedies
Valerian (*Valeriana officinalis*), Hops (*Humulus lupulus*), Jamaican Dogwood (*Piscidia erythrina*).

Homoeopathy

A good standby is Nelson's Nocturna, available in health food shops and some chemists. Listed below are some remedies which are commonly used for insomnia. They are best used short-term. If the problem persists, consider constitutional practitioner treatment.

Nux vom: For sleeplessnes after mental strain and overwork or after over-indulgence in food or alcohol. Irritability.

Coffea: Mind very active.

Rhus tox: Very restless, with aches and pains.

Arnica: Overtired. Bed feels hard.

Arsenicum: Great anguish. Restlessness of mind and body.

Nutrition

Common causes are adrenal exhaustion and hypoglycaemia, where a drop in blood sugar can cause wakefulness and anxiety. Insomnia is generally helped by improving calcium levels (hence the tradition of a milky drink before bed) and magnesium levels; also B vitamins.

GENITO/URINARY TRACT

The natural process of hormonal winding-down is the primary influence behind changes which occur in the vagina and bladder during and beyond menopause. The changes—thinning of wall lining and shrinking, loss of muscle tone and vaginal lubrication—do not cause problems for everyone, but the less fortunate can experience vaginal dryness, painful intercourse, even inflammation, bladder infections and incontinence.

Those women whose adrenal function is weak are probably more likely to experience problems arising from vaginal and bladder changes. The chief culprits, as far as depletion of the adrenal glands is concerned, are acute or prolonged stress and the overuse of stimulants such as alcohol and coffee. The strength of the kidneys should also be taken into account when looking at genito/urinary tract problems, as they have the role of regulating the fluid and hormonal balance in the body. The structural integrity of the vagina and bladder may also be affected by pregnancy, childbirth surgery, drugs, tension and other physical conditions.

Adrenal exhaustion, impaired kidney function and loss of structural integrity need not be permanent—holistic healing methods encourage the re-building and healthy maintenance of these functions, in addition to relieving symptoms. Conventional treatment of the problems includes antibiotics and HRT, which can help. However, they have drawbacks, are undesirable for many and leave the underlying causes untreated.

Vaginal Problems

The final curtain has not come down on a fulfilling sex life if your vagina is dry. Lack of lubrication is normally a sign of diminished body fluids and can safely be helped with holistic methods. Simply drinking more plain water is effective—see section on Skin and Hair changes. The use of KY jelly—a water soluble lubricant obtainable in chemists—is of great value when intercourse is uncomfortable.

Exercise promotes healthy vaginal functioning. An active sex life or failing that, self-stimulation, is a good way to maintain tone and lubrication in the pelvic area.

Pelvic floor exercises—the same as those recommended after having a baby—done regularly also help to tone and tighten the vagina. To practise them, pull in the vaginal muscles tightly, hold for a few seconds, release, then repeat. The same movement can be speeded up—rapidly tightening and releasing the muscles. Many healing yoga postures can help to strengthen the kidneys and pelvic area generally.

Some women experience irritation and inflammation of the vagina. It is worth investigating allergy or increased sensitivity as a possible factor. Typical offenders are perfumed soaps, bath products, deodorants, tampons, contraceptives and tights.

Aromatherapy
Loss of elasticity and dryness of the vagina:
Add the following quantities of drops to a bath: Geranium (2), Clary sage (2) and Sandalwood (2).

Body oil blend: Rose Maroc (10), Geranium (5), Clary Sage (5) and Sandalwood (5) in 50ml of almond oil.

Blend for long-term use: in a 10ml dropper bottle mix Geranium (35), Rose Maroc (75), Clary sage (35) and Sandalwood (35). Add 8 drops to a bath and 30 drops to 50ml of almond oil to massage twice daily into the abdomen, hips and buttocks.

Herbal Remedies
Chasteberry (*Vitex agnus castus*) to help balance the hormones.
Dry vagina: False Unicorn Root (*Chamaelirium luteum*).
Loss of Elasticity: Golden Seal (*Hydrastis*).

Homoeopathy
Loss of elasticity, dryness of the vagina
Sepia (see chapter 11 Homoeopathy). Dosage: 1 30c pill taken at night. Review and repeat if necessary.

Natural Progesterone

Used intravaginally, this may help to maintain vaginal moisture. Seek practitioner advice.

Nutrition

Loss of elasticity and dryness of the vagina

This can be due to deficiencies of vitamin E, GLA, B vitamins. Local applications of vitamin E and Aloe vera can help.

STRESS AND URGE INCONTINENCE

The passing of a small amount of urine when coughing, sneezing, running, lifting or laughing is described as stress incontinence and, together with the frequent desire to pass water (urge incontinence), is a very common problem. The main reason is loss of muscle tone. At menopause, the changing hormonal picture has an influence, but there are other factors—pregnancy, childbirth and surgery—which may also cause the pelvic floor muscles to weaken. Pelvic floor exercise (see above) are beneficial to those suffering from stress or urge incontinence. One which is particularly useful, but which might take a little practice to perfect, is to pull in the muscles while passing water to stop the flow. Hold for a few seconds, release and repeat as many times as you can.

In some women, incontinence can be aggravated by bladder irritants. Likely offenders are alcohol, caffeine, sugar, an excess of citrus and acid fruits, e.g. strawberries, pineapple and juices, chilli pepper and strong spices, all nightshade family vegetables (particularly raw), ice-cream, cold drinks and cold food. Excess liquids can also aggravate incontinence.

Aromatherapy
Body oil blend: add the following quantities of drops to 50ml of almond oil: Lavender (20), Rosemary (5), Cypress (5) and White thyme (5). Massage into the abdomen, hips and buttocks twice daily.

Herbal Remedies
Horsetail (*Equisetum*).

Homoeopathy
Causticum. Dosage: Take 1 30c pill at night. Review and repeat if necessary.

Nutrition
If the problem is loss of structural integrity in the tissues, nutrients that help connective tissues are useful: vitamin C, magnesium with calcium, silica, vitamin A and D, manganese. If it is due to infection, then cranberry juice or powder can help.

CYSTITIS

Cystitis is an inflammation of the bladder lining. The condition can be acute or chronic (recurrent) and infection may or may not be present. Attacks which persistently recur usually do so because a previous acute condition has not cleared up completely. The symptoms are an increased need to pass water and pain when passing water. There may also be blood in the urine.

There are many causative and predisposing factors which may precipitate an attack of cystitis. The underlying problem is often connected with the reproductive organs. Where there is an infection, it has normally occurred as a result of germs passing from the anus to the urethra (the tube which leads out of the bladder.) Medical treatment consists of a course of antibiotics, which, as most people are now aware, deplete the immune system. An attack of thrush, also a predisposing factor in cystitis, often follows. A situation could then develop where the sufferer is caught up in a vicious cycle of thrush and cystitis. Antibiotics usually work quickly, but they do not prevent a recurrence of cystitis.

Note If a urinary infection spreads to the kidneys, it can be very dangerous; consult a medical practitioner without delay if you develop a fever, headache and lower back pain and/or blood in the urine.

Self-help Measures and General Nutritional Advice

Act the moment any symptoms are felt, in an effort to prevent the problem spreading from the urethra into the bladder. Aim to flush it away by drinking plenty of pure hot water—at least half a pint every hour—and continue until symptoms subside. Drink home-made barley water and mix cranberry powder with water (follow instructions on the packet).

Note Cranberry juices often have added sugar—avoid these.

Other helpful liquids include coconut, aloe vera or pomegranate juice, and teas made with the herbs chamomile, coriander, lemon grass, fennel and spearmint. A warm bath can help relieve the pain. Attention should be paid to personal hygiene; avoid strong soaps, detergents, vaginal deodorants or perfumes. Tampon strings help to spread bacteria. Avoid tight clothing and nylon underwear, which increase the heat in the genital area.

Cystitis often develops after sex; reduce sexual activity and be mindful of the sexual hygiene of yourself and your partner. Contraceptive devices, e.g. the diaphragm (Dutch cap) and spermicidal creams can cause problems.

Avoid: sugar, carbonated drinks, alcohol, coffee, animal fats, eggs, starchy foods, citrus fruits and juices, strawberries, tomatoes and hot spices. Aim to keep the bloodstream clean by eating a healthy diet. Avoid becoming constipated— ensure you have plenty of fibre and water. Reduce stress, relax and rest.

Aromatherapy

Add the following quantities of drops to a bath: Eucalyptus (2), Bergamot (2) and Sandalwood (2). Use daily until the pain has eased, along with a body oil blend made with Lavender (15), Roman or Blue Chamomile (15) and Bergamot (10) in 50ml of almond oil. Use this daily on the abdomen, hips and buttocks. Also, boil half a litre of water and allow to cool before putting into a glass bottle with Chamomile (75) and Sandalwood (25). Shake thoroughly before use, then soak a fresh piece of cotton wool in a little of the solution and bathe the urethral opening after each visit to the lavatory. Take 2 garlic perles 3 times a day as an internal antibiotic.

Herbal Remedies

Marshmallow root (*Althaea officinalis*), Echinacea tincture.

Homoeopathy

Causticum: Very sensitive to cold.

Cantharis: Burning, frequency and urgency.

Staphysagria: Frequency, burning, pain before and after passing urine, no pain while passing.

Equisetum: Constant urge to urinate, passing urine does not relieve urge.

Dosage: 1 30c pill. Review and repeat if necessary.

HEADACHES

Headaches during menopause are normally associated with other symptoms, such as heavy periods, digestive disorders and constipation, tension, anxiety and depression, hot flushes and PMS. Nutritional causes include deficiency of B vitamins, hypoglycaemia, candida, toxicity of the system, food sensitivity or allergies.

Headaches are linked with so many problems that the causes can be very difficult to pinpoint. However, if you have a headache it is most likely to be stress-related. Unfortunately, the modern answer is usually to take some painkillers and carry on as before. This masks the underlying cause, which remains unresolved. Life is no longer so simple that stress can be avoided, but the likelihood of tension headaches developing can be reduced by adopting a more relaxed attitude to life.

Self-help Measures

- Allow time for regular relaxation or meditation. A useful visualisation for stress headaches is to visualise your head as a volcano, seeing problems being blown out of the top of your head.
- Curative yoga postures will help.
- Enjoy a massage or some relaxing healing. Shiatsu treatment may help.
- Try some Flower Remedies that correspond with your mood and personality.
- Eat a healthy diet; avoid stimulants.
- Try applying an ice pack to the forehead or the base of the skull at the same time as having a hot footbath, to normalise the vascular system.

Note If you are experiencing persistent headaches or they occur in conjunction with other symptoms, such as vomiting, dizziness or vision problems, seek medical help.

Aromatherapy
Make an aromatic bath using 6–8 drops of Lavender oil. Apply 1 drop of neat peppermint oil to the temples, avoiding the eyes, and 1 drop to the base of the skull with firm finger and thumb pressure up into the bone.

Herbal Remedies
Skullcap (*Scutellaria*), Cramp Bark (*Viburnum opulus*), Feverfew (*Tanacetum parthenium*).

Homoeopathy
The constitutional remedy is the best choice. There is normally no quick fix for a headache. However, self-help remedy selection can be tried, often with success. Remember, when exploring suitable remedies, to take into account the type of headache e.g. nervous, sick or congestive. Also consider the likely causes, e.g. stress, digestive disorder, and under what circumstances or when it feels better or worse.

Brief details of some remedies which are useful for headaches are given below: Take 1 30c tablet, 3 doses with 10-minute intervals between each dose.

Belladonna: Associated with heat. Rapid violent onset, restlessness, head throbs, face feels hot and is flushed bright red. Sensitivity to light. Worse: for movement, noise, lying down, bright light, cold and draughts. Better: for warmth, being upright. Belladonna can be given for hot flushes where there is restlessness and the face is very red.

Bryonia: Individual often feels stressed, irritable. There may also be constipation. Pains are sharp. Worse: for any motion, touch, warmth, eating. Better: for pressure, being alone, cold, rest.

Nux Vomica: Headaches are associated with tension, nausea, digestive disturbance, constipation or effects of over-indulgence in food or alcohol. Extremely irritable, critical, nervous. Worse: in the morning, from coldness, noise, stimulants and rich foods. Better: from warmth, damp weather, firm pressure, for a nap, rest, in the evening.

Pulsatilla: Headaches occur as a result of stress, digestive disturbance, constipation, after eating rich food, associated with problems arising from hormonal changes. Type is inclined to weep, moods change quickly. Worse: from heat and stuffy rooms, in the evening, after eating. Better: in the fresh air, cold applications, cold food and drink, from sympathy and affection.

Natural Progesterone

Natural progesterone may be of help. Seek practitioner advice first.

MENSTRUAL IRREGULARITIES

VARIABLE CYCLE

Changes in the pattern of menstruation are among the first signs that hormone levels are fluctuating and that menopause is drawing near. The monthly cycle and the duration of the periods may lengthen or shorten, and there could be an increase or decrease in blood loss.

The effects of menstrual changes at menopause vary from woman to woman. For some, their periods fade out gradually, posing no problem; for others they stop suddenly—although this is unusual. Many women face difficulties as a result of an erratic cycle, prolonged or heavy bleeding.

Aromatherapy

Add the following quantities of drops to a bath: Lavender (4), Basil (1), White Thyme (1) and Geranium (2).

Body oil blend: 24 drops in 50ml of sweet almond oil— Lavender (12), Basil (3), White Thyme (3) and Geranium (6). Use for at least 2-3 full cycles.

Blend for long-term use: in a 10ml dropper bottle mix 80 drops of Lavender, Basil (20), Thyme (20), Geranium (50). Add 6-8 drops to a bath and 30 drops to 50ml of sweet almond oil and use to massage into the abdomen, buttocks and hips. Use for at least 2-3 full cycles.

Homoeopathy

Selection of the constitutional remedy is the correct approach. (Specific remedies are mentioned under Pain and Fibroids.)

Herbal Remedies

Chasteberry (*Vitex agnus castus*), Yarrow (*Achillea millefolium*) and Thuja occidentalis are useful herbs for the menstrual function generally.

HEAVY BLEEDING (MENORRHAGIA)

Hormonal imbalance and the presence of fibroids are the two most common reasons for heavy bleeding. Both conditions can be helped by holistic healing methods. Many other causes of heavy bleeding require specific medical care and it is advisable, if you are experiencing heavy or prolonged bleeding, to obtain an early medical opinion.

Note Always seek medical advice if your menstrual cycle is less than 21 days, if bleeding occurs between periods or after they have ceased.

Aromatherapy
Excessive bleeding and fibroids
Add the following quantities of drops to a bath: Cypress (2), Geranium (2), Lemon (1) and Lavender (3).

Body oil blend: 25 drops in 50ml of sweet almond oil—Geranium (8), Rose (10) and Lemon (7). Use for at least 2–3 full cycles.

Blend for long-term use: in a 10ml dropper bottle mix Cypress (50), Geranium (50), Lemon (25) and Lavender (60), and add 6–8 drops to a bath.

Herbal Remedies
Lady's Mantle (*Alchemilla vulgaris*) and Shepherd's Purse (*Capsella bursa-pastoris*).

Nutrition
It is wise to take an iron supplement, as heavy/prolonged bleeding can result in iron deficiency. The commonly prescribed non-organic iron can cause constipation or diarrhoea, so it is best to try a more organic form of iron, which is obtainable from health food shops. Normal dosages are 10mg a day, but higher ones may be necessary during very heavy periods. It is easy to take an excess of iron, so have levels checked regularly if you are supplementing a great deal.

For those not wishing to eat meat, substantial quantities of iron are found in fresh red fish—salmon, tuna—shellfish; dulse and other sea vegetables; red vegetables—beetroot, red cabbage—and apricots. Avoid foods from the nightshade family if you are anaemic.

PAINFUL PERIODS (DYSMENORRHOEA)

Painful periods often relate to problems with liver function. Other factors which could have a bearing on this problem include: hormone imbalance, fibroids, endometriosis, candida, postural problems, dietary deficiencies, depletion and tension. If you are in any doubt, it is best to consult a practitioner.

Self-help Measures

- Eat a nutritious, low-fat diet.
- Have plenty of regular exercise.
- The warmth from a hot water bottle laid on the abdomen can be very soothing.
- Look at ways which will help you to relax (see Chapter Fifteen).
- There are many curative yoga postures for menstrual disorders.

Aromatherapy

Mix the following drops in 2 teaspoons of sweet almond oil: Roman Chamomile (2), Clary sage (2) and Lavender (3) and massage the abdomen, buttocks, hips and the tops of the thighs. Apply warm compresses with 2 drops of each of the above oils.

Herbal Remedies

Viburnum prunifolium and Anemone pulsatilla.

Homoeopathy

Mag. phos.: suited to the slim, nervous type, dark complexion. Cramping of muscles with radiating pain; exhaustion. Worse: at night, for cold air, water, touch, motion, right side. Better: from warmth, pressure, bending double.

Colocynthis: suited to the irritable type. Painful cramps with all pains. Worse: evening, anger, after eating. Better: from coffee, bending double, hard pressure. Dosage: 1 30c pill taken at night. Review and repeat if necessary.

Nutrition

The B vitamins, in particular Niacin (B3) and Pyridoxine (B6), are known to help. The correct levels of magnesium and calcium, vitamin E, iron and essential fatty acids should be maintained. Include the following in your diet: turmeric, asafoetida, ginger, nutmeg (a small amount only) and natural liquorice. A warm sesame oil massage of the abdomen can ease the pain.

FIBROIDS AND HYSTERECTOMY

Uterine fibroids are growths which can vary from being almost undetectable to the size of a grapefruit. They are rarely malignant. The condition is a symptom of hormonal imbalance and congestion in the body. Following menopause, in the environment of a changed hormonal picture, fibroids are inclined to shrink and are less of a problem. However, many women become anaemic and debilitated as a result of heavy and prolonged bleeding associated with the growth of fibroids.

The most commonly proposed medical solution is a partial hysterectomy—the removal of the womb (and sometimes one ovary). In fact, it is the main reason for this form of surgery. Partial hysterectomy carried out before menopause can result in premature menopausal symptoms being experienced, though it is more likely for any symptoms to arise only when menopause occurs. This is not so, however, in the case of a full hysterectomy, which involves the removal of both ovaries in addition to the womb. The sudden shock to the hormonal system plunges a woman straight into menopause, often resulting in further, quite severe symptoms, for which synthetic hormonal treatment is normally prescribed.

Holistic methods may be successfully used to help relieve symptoms following a hysterectomy. The possibility of emotional factors being involved in the development of fibroids should not be overlooked. The seeds can be sown by any number of emotions—past hurts, anger, resentment, dissatisfaction and problems relating to unexplored femininity or creativity. Practitioner help may be considered, by way of counselling, hands-on healing and other holistic therapies. Personal awareness could be explored on a self-help basis, together with meditation/visualisation, Bach Remedies and other methods discussed earlier.

The causes and treatment of fibroids are complex and it is advisable to see a practitioner. Once again, the good health of the liver is important as is pelvic circulation to relieve congestion. My personal experience is that fibroids respond well to macrobiotic dietary treatment and Traditional Chinese Medicine.

Aromatherapy
See blends for heavy bleeding.

Natural Progesterone
If you are receiving Natural Progesterone treatment for fibroids, a useful self-help measure is to take a liver tonic as well.

NERVOUS PROBLEMS

Menopause is a time when hormones are changing; the adrenal glands and liver are endeavouring to adapt. If there are factors preventing a smooth transition, such as stress, deep-seated emotional blocks, unsatisfactory lifestyle and nutritional deficiencies, nervous problems can result. Do not be alarmed or ashamed if you are suffering in this respect; there are many avenues where help may be obtained, both holistically and along more conventional lines.

Conventional methods recognise that psychosomatic disease is a reality—what is going on inside the mind can also affect the body. The possibility that this could work the other way round is now also gaining acceptance—that physical illness and environmental factors have a greater effect on the mind and emotions than previously envisaged. Holistic methods of healing see all symptoms in an individual—physical, mental and emotional—as being inextricably linked.

When exploring holistic self-help measures to overcome nervous problems, first look at what might be the cause, e.g. stress, hormonal changes, poor diet or other dietary factors, chemical toxicity, lack of regular exercise or relaxation. The solution may be simply a case of improving the diet, talking to someone willing to listen, making minor adjustments to your lifestyle, trying Flower Remedies, having a healing, using specific yoga healing postures or asking a friend for a massage.

Herbal Remedies
Chasteberry (*Vitex agnus castus*), Lavender (*Lavendula officinalis*), Rosemary (*Rosmarinus officinalis*), Betony (*Stachys betonica*).

Homoeopathy
Treatment should be directed to the constitutional remedy. Aconite (in higher potency, 200c) can be used for any of the conditions under Nervous Problems, where the person is very fearful.

Nutrition
Nervous problems can be easily balanced with a harmonic way of eating. For instance, too much meat in the diet may produce tension, stress, irritability or anxiety, while an excess of sugar could produce hyperactivity or moody behaviour.

Depression, mood swings, irritability, anxiety or panic and lack of concentration can all relate to hypoglycaemia and/or the effects of candida overgrowth. Adrenal and nervous system exhaustion and depletion of nutrients that feed them are also possible causes. Mood swings can be caused by food sensitivity (allergy). Depression can also relate to liver congestion, which can be helped with aloe vera juice and lecithin, and the diet recommended for cooling hot flushes. Deficiencies of B vitamins, magnesium and calcium should also be investigated.

Memory problems or lack of concentration can improve with B vitamins, lecithin (or the active ingredients of choline and inositol), CoQ10, ginkgo biloba. The supplement Phosphatidyl serine magnesium is useful for supporting the adrenals, nervous system and memory.

DEPRESSION

It is quite normal to feel sad from time to time. Most people say they feel better after a good cry, then bounce back into life again. True depression is less transient and has clinically recognised symptoms, both mental and physical. Common symptoms of depression include:

- fatigue not relieved by rest or sleep
- apathy
- lethargy
- low self-esteem
- feeling of desolation
- pessimistic and irrational thoughts (can feel suicidal)
- disturbed sleep
- loss of appetite or eating when not hungry.

There are a multitude of reasons why depression might develop. It is also true that some people, by virtue of inherited tendencies or social circumstances, are at greater risk than others. However, changing hormone levels during menopause can cause some women to be affected by depression for the first time in their lives. While frightening and distressing in itself, depression may seem particularly hard to deal with in the mid-life years, when there may be other health problems, major new experiences and feelings to contend with. They may include:

- grief and shock as a result of children leaving home, followed by feelings of emptiness and having no useful purpose
- fear of being too old to be offered work
- a partner's declining desire to make love, contributing to feelings of being 'over the hill' and unattractive
- the increased possibility of having to care for elderly parents—even being faced with their death.

Conventional ways of treating depression have their place, but do not go far enough towards addressing the causes. The use of drugs, whilst bringing relief in the short-term, carries the risk of dependency and side-effects. The possibility that you are depressed or that depression might lie beneath other symptoms of ill-health may not have occurred to you. Whatever the circumstances, don't wait, hoping it will go away. Take steps to obtain an early diagnosis—it's best to know exactly what you are dealing with. Find someone in whom you feel safe to confide—a friend, family member or counsellor. A therapist will treat your problem with confidentiality, make an assessment of the situation and your needs, encouraging your participation in the process of healing.

Regular exercise can be very uplifting—explore what might suit you. Explore relaxation methods—yoga, meditation, breathing techniques, massage. Healing is very relaxing. Be kind to yourself, make a point of doing something every day which will give you pleasure, and keep a diary of your progress and feelings. Painting and art therapy may appeal to you as a means of expression.

Eat a wholesome diet. Oats nourish and strengthen the whole system. They have long been used to help depression and nervous debility. St. John's Wort (Hypericum perforatum) is also an old remedy for depression and associated exhaustion.

Depression does not have to be dealt with alone; there are a lot of people out there who will be prepared to give you their time and help you build the confidence and determination needed to reach the light at the end of the tunnel.

Aromatherapy

Add the following quantities of drops to a bath: Grapefruit (2), Bergamot (2) and Geranium (3).

Body oil blend: Rose (8), Bergamot (6), Tangerine (5) and Geranium (6) in 50ml of almond oil.

Blend of drops for long-term use: in a 10ml dropper bottle mix Grapefruit (50), Bergamot (50), Geranium (75) and add 6 drops to a bath.

Bach Remedies

Dr Bach placed 6 remedies in the group 'despondency and despair'.

- Larch: As a type, despondent, lacks confidence, anticipates failure, feels inferior. The mood may descend following an accident, shock, severe illness. Often needs a supporting fear remedy.
- Elm: Normally a confident type, can become overwhelmed with burden of responsibility, resulting in feelings of inadequacy and despondency. State is normally temporary.
- Pine: Full of self reproach and guilt which is buried deep inside. Always apologising. Becomes depressed at not being able to live up to own high ideals.
- Crab Apple: Often associated with Pine, the individual feels self-hatred, despair, uncleanliness.
- Star of Bethlehem: Shock in any form, including unsuspected delayed effects. Grief and sorrow.
- Sweet Chestnut: Extreme anguish, hopelessness and despair. Feels as though limit of endurance reached. Does not tend towards suicide as Cherry Plum might. Types who might eventually need Sweet Chestnut are Oak, Vervain, Agrimony, Centaury.

Among other remedies which might be considered are:

- Cherry Plum: Fears mind might give way, desperation, deep depression, irrational thoughts—could feel suicidal.
- Olive: Total fatigue of mind and body, everything is an effort.
- Gorse: Extreme pessimism and hopelessness, gives up without trying. Not forthcoming.
- Gentian: Depression due to a setback from a known cause. Doubts situation will improve.
- White Chestnut: Worries go round and round in the mind.
- Mustard: Feelings of deep gloom which descend suddenly and lift just as suddenly — without apparent reason.

Natural Progesterone
Natural progesterone may be of help. Seek practitioner advice first.

ANXIETY, FEARFUL AND IRRATIONAL THOUGHTS, PANIC ATTACKS, MOOD SWINGS, IRRITABILITY

The body is designed in such a way that it can raise its tempo and deal with emergency 'fight or flight' situations, then return quickly and smoothly to normal functioning. Anxiety is a key red alert body/mind message that you have been placed under some form of threat or stress and are finding it difficult to cope and maintain a balanced state. The response of anxiety can cause mental and physical symptomatic repercussions to occur throughout the body. Reactions could be numerous—symptoms in turn causing other symptoms: panic attacks, palpitations, headaches, dry mouth, flushing, dizziness, raised blood pressure, insomnia, diarrhoea, sexual problems. In addition, there may be the sort of symptoms often attributed to PMS, including fluctuating moods, weepiness, irritability, depression, lack of confidence and irrational thoughts.

There are no quick solutions to nervous problems in menopause. When these are deep-seated, trying to unravel and release past hurts which reveal themselves during this period might involve time and much hard work on personal awareness issues or cooperation with a professional counsellor. Making lifestyle changes and perhaps embarking on a very different way of eating from what you have been used to for the past forty to fifty years is equally challenging and time-consuming. Determination, willpower and patience may be needed before benefits are observed.

If you are suffering from anxiety and other nervous problems and wish to try holistic self-help, use the general guidance given on diet, relaxation, meditation and healing to build a foundation for your personal programme. In addition, you might try sharing your anxiety with those who are willing to listen. Also consider yoga, or T'ai-chi, and breathing exercises. Take some form of exercise daily. Other suggestions include hand and foot massage, a back massage using a body massage oil blend, drinking calming herbal teas such as chamomile, limeflower and valerian (also available as tablets from health food shops).

Eat regular meals—the spirits fall when you are hungry. Reduce or exclude excess protein and fats and sugary foods if you are experiencing mood swings, irritability and exhaustion as too many will lower blood sugar.

Aromatherapy

Anxiety and Irritability: Add 4 drops each of Lavender and Petitgrain to a warm bath.

Body oil blend: The following drops in 50ml of almond oil: Petitgrain (8), Neroli (10) and Lavender (8).

If very panicky and hysterical, add Vetivert (2), Neroli (2) and Chamomile Maroc (2) to a bath and afterwards massage 1 drop of Vetivert anti-clockwise into the solar plexus.

Mood swings Add Geranium (4) and Lavender (4) to a bath.

Body oil blend: Lavender (12), Petitgrain (10) and Geranium (8) in 50ml of almond oil.

Fear and irrational thoughts Add the following quantities of drops to a bath: Sandalwood (3), Ylang ylang (2) and Frankincense (2).

Body oil blend: Ylang ylang (6) Petitgrain (10) and Rose (8) in 50ml of almond oil.

Blend for long-term use: in a 10ml dropper bottle mix Sandalwood (75), Ylang ylang (50) and Frankincense (50) and add 6–8 drops to a bath.

Bach Remedies

- Mimulus: Anxiety and nervousness; known fears.
- Vervain: Nervous tension and stress.
- Red Chestnut: Natural worrier. Anxious about family. Imagines the worst.
- White Chestnut: Worries go round and round in the mind.
- Impatiens: Nervous, irritable and impatient.
- Walnut: Oversensitivity.
- Scleranthus: Changeability—mood swings. Useful with any form of imbalance.
- Mustard: Deep gloom descends suddenly then lifts just as

suddenly for no apparent reason. Useful for premenstrual blues and mood swings.
- Rock Rose: Panic and terror—known fears.
- Aspen: Anxiety, apprehension which has no logical explanation. Can panic.
- Cherry Plum: When emotional control is lost; irrational and suicidal thoughts.

Homoeopathy
Panic attacks: Aconite where there is fear present, or Ignatia where there is emotional distress. Take 1 200c pill.

FORGETFULNESS, LACK OF CONCENTRATION AND CONFUSION

Becoming forgetful, losing concentration or feeling confused during menopause might prompt the fear that you are in the early stages of senile dementia. This is very unlikely to be the case. There are numerous reasons why these symptoms occur, including side-effects from tranquillisers and sleeping pills, or nutritional deficiencies. They may also be a symptom of other conditions, e.g. candida, hypoglycaemia and M.E.

In Traditional Chinese Medicine, lack of concentration and confusion is usually attributed to spleen disharmony; and forgetfulness to kidney essence deficiency. There is also the possibility that a body/mind message is being broadcast and that a break or a holiday might be all that is needed to get back to normal. Perhaps the less logical, creative side of your brain could be used to greater benefit. Ask yourself whether there is another job you would rather do, a creative hobby or pursuit there hasn't been time for, or something you would like to study. A woman's changing role in mid-life presents an ideal opportunity to consider making rewarding changes.

Aromatherapy

Inhale 1 drop each of Basil, Rosemary and Peppermint from a tissue.

Bach Remedies

- Clematis: Inability to concentrate, loss of memory, day-dreaming.
- Wild Oat: Uncertain of direction in life.

LOSS OF LIBIDO

There is no foundation for the belief that your sex drive automatically declines at menopause. Quite the reverse can be true! However, a loss of interest in sex *can* be a problem for some women. Many factors could be involved, such as depletion of the kidneys and adrenal exhaustion, vaginal dryness, fatigue, a partner's sexual problems, relationship difficulties, underlying depression, lifestyle, poor diet, sleep, exercise, stress. If there is a depletion in health, the body will take protective action to ensure energy is conserved for healing purposes rather than allow it to be expended in sexual activity. A healthy sex life depends very much on adrenal good health. Depleted adrenal function can be behind many problems likely to influence libido.

Aromatherapy

Add the following quantities of drops to a bath: Ylang ylang (1), Rose (2), Patchouli (2) and Sandalwood (2).

Body oil blend: Ylang ylang (4), Rose (10), Patchouli (6) and Sandalwood (6) in 50ml of almond oil.

Blend for long-term use: in a 10ml dropper bottle mix Ylang ylang (30), Rose (50), Patchouli (50) and Sandalwood (50) and add 6–8 drops to a bath and 30 drops to 50ml almond oil for the body.

Herbal Remedies
Oats (*Avena sativa*), Damiana (*Turnera diffusa*), Rosemary (*Rosmarinus officinalis*) Siberian Ginseng (*Eluetherococcus*).

SKIN AND HAIR CHANGES

There are many factors which influence the condition of the skin and two of its appendages, the hair and nails. Inherited tendencies, lifestyle and the choice of skin care products may have a bearing, but the chief factor governing skin condition comes from within. This means the overall health of the body—how it is nourished, both physically and emotionally, and how well it is functioning.

Various natural skin changes occur as a woman ages and she passes through the change of life. These could result in dry skin, loss of skin tone and the development of wrinkles. Facial hair may start to grow, or hair could be lost from the head and other parts of the body.

Holistic methods are of great value in the prevention and treatment of problems of this nature, as they encourage the re-balancing of the body's nutritional, hormonal and emotional health. In traditional terms, the skin, hair and nails are affected by the health and action of certain organs in the body with which they have a working relationship. For example, most people have seen how their skin glows after energetic exercise, when the lungs have been fully utilised and the circulation stimulated.

The skin, in addition to its protective, balancing role is an organ of elimination. If any of the other organs of elimination are depleted, then the skin will be required to do more work. If this is the case, there is a strong likelihood that it will throw out symptoms of protest. The inclusion of too much fat in the diet is more readily associated with a greasy skin, but it can also make the skin and hair very dry. When excess fat collects under the skin, it forms a barrier, precluding natural moisture from reaching the surface. If your skin is dry and itchy, an excess of fat and white flour products might be the simple cause. Dry skin can also result when there is not enough fat in the diet, while dry, brittle hair may be a sign that the kidneys are depleted.

Self-help

Dietary quality is the first thing to check when investigating skin problems. Try to maintain a balanced, wholefood diet with plenty of vegetables and fruit. Include as much organic food as possible. (See the guidelines in Chapter Thirteen Nutrition and Diet.)

As we age, more fluid is naturally lost from the body. This could result in dehydration affecting internal functions as well as the surface of the skin, making it dry and causing it to look older. Avoid fluids which have a dehydrating effect. Drinking plain water is the most effective way of replenishing fluids. Avoid smoking. It has an ageing effect on the skin and depletes the body of vitamin C.

Look after adrenal health. Oestrogen, which helps to maintain body fluid levels, is increasingly produced by the adrenal glands from menopause onwards. Have plenty of exercise. If you feel that stress might have something to do with your skin problems or hair loss, set aside time for relaxation—many suggestions and techniques are given in this book.

Chemicals and synthetic substances can play havoc with the skin, hair and nails. They are now so bound up with modern living that avoiding them is difficult. The ingredients in many mass-market skin care products can include harsh detergents, chemicals and synthetic substances. Gentle, natural skin care preparations and cosmetics which have not been tested on animals can be obtained in specialist outlets like the Body Shop, health food shops and some chemists. Look for ranges which have been specially formulated for the mature skin.

DRY SKIN AND HAIR

Aromatherapy

Dry Skin Add the following quantities of drops to a bath: Geranium (2), Patchouli (2) and Sandalwood (2).

Body oil blend: 26 drops in 50ml of almond oil: Geraniuim (10), Patchouli (8) and Sandalwood (8).

Blend of drops for long-term use: in a 10ml dropper bottle mix Geranium (50), Patchouli (65) and Sandalwood (65) and add 6–8 drops to a bath and 30 drops to 50ml of almond oil. Also add Rose (5) or Jasmine (5) and Sandalwood (5) to an unperfumed night cream, and Geranium (3), Sandalwood (3) and Rose (3) to a day cream or jojoba.

Dry Hair Add the following quantities of drops to 50ml jojoba: Sandalwood (9), Ylang ylang (7), Geranium (7) and Cedarwood (8). Massage into scalp and hair then wrap in clingfilm and a warm towel for 30 minutes. You will need to shampoo twice, first with undiluted shampoo; then condition as usual.

Nutrition

Avoid all kinds of sugars, fats and oils (particularly heated), fried, greasy, oily foods, raw salt on food, stimulants (alcohol, coffee, tea, colas) which also have a dehydrating effect on the body, spices, cold/frozen foods, eggs, cheese, meat.

Take burdock or dandelion tea, aloe vera (internally and

as an external application). Rub skin with white cabbage juice. Look for deficiencies of vitamin A, B, and essential fatty acids. Take GLA in the form of Evening Primrose oil or linseed oil.

BRITTLE NAILS
The mineral silica will help to strengthen nails. Silica is obtainable from health food stores in tissue salt or homoeopathic form. The herb horsetail is a rich source of this mineral.

Aromatherapy
Add the following quantities of drops to 50ml of mixed almond oil and jojoba: Patchouli (8), Sandalwood (8) and Lavender (7). Pour a little into a small bowl and soak nails for 20 minutes. Remove most of the excess and massage residue into hands and nails.

HAIR LOSS AND GROWTH OF UNWANTED HAIR
When women are deficient in progesterone, they manufacture more male hormones. This can lead to hair loss, together with the growth of unwanted facial and body hair. The whole picture of hormonal balance should be looked at.

Homoeopathy
The constitutional remedy is best in respect of skin and hair changes. Sepia can be of use to help thinning hair.

Natural Progesterone
Natural progesterone may be of benefit. Seek practitioner advice first.

Nutrition

Look for possible nutritional deficiency, especially of vitamins D and B, zinc and GLA.

WATER RETENTION

Retention of fluid in the body is a very common condition and can have many causes. If the organs involved in the elimination of waste matter in the body are sluggish or blocked, water retention may be one of the resulting symptoms. This is not as worrying as it sounds. Given the appropriate holistic care and time, these organs are quite capable of self-regeneration to the point where normal functioning is again achieved.

The simple healthy practice of drinking plain water has almost vanished in everyday life, while tea, coffee and fizzy drinks—many of which contain caffeine—are drunk to excess. These are nowhere near as effective as water either in quenching the thirst or maintaining correct body fluid balance, so necessary for cell renewal and efficient waste elimination.

Tea and coffee are both diuretics. Coffee has a particularly unbalancing effect on the body's hydration system—its powerful action causing essential vitamins and minerals to be lost from the system. Swollen legs and ankles are often experienced during menopause, and might also occur pre-menstrually. Self-help could start with taking regular exercise, avoiding prolonged standing and resting with the legs elevated above head height for at least 15 minutes daily.

In addition to drinking plenty of plain water every day, you should eat a balanced, wholefood diet, reducing your intake of sweet foods, fats, salt and salty foods (excess salt encourages water retention and stresses the kidneys).

Fluid retention can be a side-effect of HRT and some sleep-inducing drugs. Chemical diuretics can adversely affect the body's mineral balance. On the other hand, there are many plants and everyday foods which have a natural, gentle diuretic action—celery, cucumber, grapes, melons, onions, carrots, green vegetables and asparagus. Dandelion, recommended below, is extremely effective as a natural diuretic. It also tones the kidneys and is particularly useful in treating pre-menstrual fluid retention. Celery, onion, asparagus and dandelion are all available as bottled plant juices.

Self-help measures can be effective in bringing relief, but if the problem or tendency persists, practitioner help should be sought.

Aromatherapy
General fluid retention Add the following quantities of drops to a bath: Lemon (1), Geranium (2) and Cypress (2).

Body oil blend: Lemon (6), Geranium (10) and Cypress (9) in 50ml of almond oil.

Swollen legs and ankles Add Geranium (2) and Rosemary (2) to a tepid footbath and soak for 20–30 minutes. Stroke legs gently in an upwards direction and around the abdomen with the following blend: Rosemary (8), Orange (10), Geranium (8) and White Thyme (2) in 50 ml almond oil.

Herbal Remedies
Dandelion leaf (*Taraxacum herba*), Yarrow (*Achillea millefolium*), Pellitory in the Wall (*Parietaria diffusa*).

Homoeopathy
Apis mel: Worse: from heat in any form, the slightest touch,

pressure, late afternoon, after sleep. Better: from cool in any form, in the open air, motion, uncovering. Dosage: 1 30c pill taken at night. Review and repeat if necessary.

Natural Progesterone
Natural progesterone may be helpful. Seek practitioner advice first.

Nutrition
In particular, check for food sensitivity (allergy) and candida overgrowth. Extra vitamin B6 in the form of pyrodoxal 5 phosphate is very useful, along with a general B complex. Vitamins D and C may also be relevant.

WEIGHT VARIATION
The build-up of unwanted fat or fluid in the body causes it to become overweight, putting the entire system under strain. Perhaps the two best-known consequences of this are high blood pressure and back pain. The battle with middle-aged spread can usually be avoided if eating habits in later life are geared to needing fewer calories to maintain body weight.

Being overweight is not always caused by overeating. There are numerous other reasons for weight gain, from the obvious—too much fatty food, water retention, inherited tendencies—to the more difficult to determine. These may include deep-seated emotional stress, hormonal/thyroid imbalance, or other functional problems best left in the hands of a practitioner.

Most overweight conditions are helped, however, by making adjustments to unhealthy eating patterns, chaotic attitudes and lifestyle.

EMOTIONAL FACTORS

Prolonged stress, dissatisfaction or a traumatic emotional experience, if harboured and not released, can manifest as either weight loss or gain—for instance, becoming thin with worry or grief is an acknowledged reaction to emotional stress. Weight gain can also arise from emotional causes or a state of mind. Over-indulgence in food (or drink) can be the result of seeking comfort in times of depression, boredom, loneliness and grief.

If you feel your weight problems could involve emotional or lifestyle issues, consider counselling, healing, Bach Remedies or constitutional homoeopathic treatment as means of help. Dieting is not the answer to being overweight. Most dieters return to their original eating habits and fail to keep their new shape for very long. Indeed, crash dieting upsets the whole metabolism, with weight being gained more easily afterwards than it was before.

The best way to lose weight, if there are no treatable underlying problems, is to adopt a healthy, new, wholefood way of eating, combined with plenty of regular exercise. Weight loss will be slow but sure; the metabolism having time to adjust slowly, thus decreasing the possibility of unwanted weight returning.

Aromatherapy

Add the following quantities of drops to a bath: Bergamot (2), Geranium (3), White Thyme (1).

Body oil blend: Bergamot (8), Geranium (12) and White Thyme (4) in 50ml of almond oil.

Blend for long-term use: in a 10ml dropper bottle mix Bergamot (70), Geranium (70) and White Thyme (30) and add 6–8 drops to a bath and 25 drops to 50ml almond oil.

Bach Remedies

Remedies for type and mood should be considered together with remedies to help with the effects of underlying trauma, e.g. shock, grief, fear, etc., if applicable.

Nutrition

Overeating is a popular pastime in wealthy nations and is one of the major causes of premature ageing. Our modern, over-rich food is responsible for most 'civilised' diseases such as obesity, cancer and mid-life onset diabetes. But overeating is by no means confined to meat-eaters. It often occurs among vegetarians who have not made a proper transition from animal foods—i.e. they transfer to lots of cheese, eggs, etc. without first cleansing the system of accumulated meat fats. They are also inclined to overeat new, lighter foods because their systems are still locked into old habits. Overeating can also be a direct result of emotional and spiritual emptiness.

GROUND RULES FOR LOSING WEIGHT AND ACHIEVING A BALANCED DIET
(for conventional people who overeat)

- Eat proper, regular meals—snacking is the first step towards weight gain.
- Take time to eat your meals. Be aware of and enjoy your food (no TV). This will put you on the right path towards correcting snacking habits.
- Chew your food well.
- Do not be rigid about your diet, but learn how to stop eating when you are two-thirds full.
- Tune in to yourself and be aware of what affects your appetite—including menstruation, ovulation and stress.

Observe when/how/what/how much (keep a diary) you are eating or drinking to be polite or out of habit.

- Avoid late meals—try to finish your last meal at least two hours before going to bed.

If you are underweight, try eating little and often but increasing your intake of hot and cooked foods (rather than too many cold, raw foods), including warming spices such as fresh ginger and cumin which help digestion. Use sesame oil which is warming and nourishing both eaten with food or used as a massage oil.

Natural Progesterone

Natural progesterone may be beneficial. Seek practitioner advice first.

Afterword

Readers may question why many holistic therapies have been omitted from this book. This is because it has not been possible to cover them all and is no reflection on the value of those that have not appeared. However, I hope enough advice *has* been given to encourage readers to explore holistic measures for themselves.

The information I have given is not intended to be prescriptive, or to suggest that readers abandon their conventional medication. It has simply offered a collection of holistic philosophy and selected therapies, with the aim of demonstrating how illness can be prevented and optimum health achieved and maintained.

Although principally aimed at a female readership within the ages of forty and sixty, I hope there has been plenty to interest and help both younger and older women. I have endeavoured to guide readers, especially those in their menopausal years, to learn of the factors which might be damaging their health and become more in touch with the needs of their body, mind and spirit. It has been my aim to help them develop new values and an understanding of the wider picture of life so that they can take charge of the management of their own health.

To remind you of its underlying message, here are a few simple checkpoints:

*   eat a healthy diet
*   avoid substances that are harmful to the body and the environment
*   remember to breathe properly and maintain good posture

- ensure you have plenty of clean, fresh air and exercise
- endeavour to avoid the trap of spending the greater part of your life feeling worried and stressed.

Bear in mind that stressful living is part of the modern world. The secret of handling it lies in your reactions and the ways you choose to make coping easier.

Perhaps the most difficult aspect of living holistically is learning the deeper understanding of symptoms and the benefits to be derived from seeking answers to the meaning behind them. It is important for healer and patient alike to recognise the causes behind symptoms, in order for complete, lasting healing to take place. Remember, the route to happiness and health is travelled from within, and it is possible to make changes in your lifestyle and eating patterns which will also affect your emotional health. Many of the case histories I have used clearly illustrate this point—showing how the holistic approach in the treatment of people and conditions can be beneficial on all levels.

As your physical well-being improves and becomes more balanced, so you will find your awareness of yourself and the world around you also moves up a gear, providing you with the impetus you need to deal with any imbalances in your emotional and spiritual life.

Everything is connected. Understanding this can help you heal yourself and your surroundings into wholeness.

Marylyn Meek

Useful Addresses

AROMATHERAPY

UK

International Federation of Aromatherapists 2–4 Chiswick High Road, London W4 1TH. Tel.: 0181 742 2605. Practitioner referrals: Send A5 sae and cheque for £2.50 with a request for their countrywide directory of aromatherapists.

Suppliers

Swanfleet Centre 93 Fortress Road, London NW5 1AG. Tel.: 0171 267 6717.

The London School of Aromatherapy is at the same address.

N. & G. Rich 2 Coval Gardens, London SW14 7DG. Tel.: 0181 878 2976.

Tisserand Newtown Road, Hove, Sussex BN3 7BA. Tel.: 01273 325666 for details of stockists.

USA

National Association for Holistic Aromatherapy PO Box 17622, Boulder, Colorado 80308-7622.

AUSTRALIA

I.F.A. (Australia) 25 Singleton Road, North Baldwin 3104, Victoria.

BACH FLOWER REMEDIES

The Bach Centre Mount Vernon, Sotwell, Wallingford, Oxon OX10 OPZ. Tel.: 01491 834678.

The Bach Centre will supply details of remedy stockists and a practitioner list.

COUNSELLING

British Association for Counselling 1 Regent Place, Rugby, Warks CV21 2PJ. Tel.: 01788 550899.

Send sae for a list of counsellors and organisations.

EASTERN MEDICINE

AYURVEDA

Ayurvedic Council of Great Britain 50 Penywern Road, London SW5 9SX. Tel.: 0171 370 2255.

Treatment and products. Telephone for local practitioner.

The Ayurvedic Trading Co. East West Centre, 10 High Street, Glastonbury BA6 9DU.

Tel./fax: 01458 833382.

Treatment and mail order service.

Ayurveda, The Practice The Manor House, Gaulby Road, Kings Norton, Leics LE7 9BA. Tel./fax: 0116 259 6633.

Treatment, training and retreats.

SHIATSU

International Shiatsu Commission 68 Fairfield Road, East Grimstead, West Sussex RH19 4HB. Tel. 01342 328240. Fax. 01342 326822.

For practitioner register and details of schools.

TRADITIONAL CHINESE MEDICINE

UK

The British Acupuncture Council Park House, 206–208 Latimer Road, London W10 6RE. Tel.: 0181 964 0222.

List of local practitioners sent free of charge.

The Register of Chinese Herbal Medicine P.O. Box 400, Wembley, Middlesex HA9 9NZ. Tel.: 0181 904 1357.

For further information and a list of countrywide practitioners send a cheque for £2.50 and an A5 sae.

Suppliers

Acumedic 101–105 Camden High Street, London NW1 7JN. Tel.: 0171 388 5783.

Remedies and dried herbs. Mail order service.

East West Herbs 3 Neal's Yard, London WC2H 9DP. Tel.: (0171) 379 1312.

Mail order service, specialising in Traditional Chinese Medicine Dispensary and prescription service. Provides practitioner details. A qualified practitioner is available to give general, informal advice.

USA

National Acupuncture and Oriental Medicine Alliance 1833 North 105th Street, Seattle, WA 98133.

AUSTRALIA

Australian Traditional Medicine Society 120 Blaxland Road, Ryde, New South Wales 2112.

YOGA

Yoga Therapy Centre Royal London Homoeopathic Hospital, 60 Great Ormond Street WC1N 3HR. Tel.: 0171 833 7267.

Will supply a list of countrywide therapists who are able to help with menopausal and menstrual problems.

HEALING

UK

The National Federation of Spiritual Healers (NFSH) Old Manor Farm Studio, Church Street, Sunbury-on-Thames, Middlesex TW16 6RG. Tel.: 01932 783164.

Healer Referral Service: Tel.: 0891 616080.

AUSTRALIA
The National Council of Australian Spiritual Healers Association P.O. Box 9187, Alice Springs, NT 0871.
Affiliated to NFSH.

HERBAL MEDICINE
UK
School of Phytotherapy (Herbal Medicine) Bodle St. Green, Nr. Hailsham, East Sussex BN27 4RJ. Tel.: 01323 833812 (referrals).
Herbline UK Tel.: 01323 832858.
A new helpline staffed by qualified medical herbalists. Hours: Tuesday, Wednesday and Friday 9.00am–3.00pm. **Note** No diagnostic advice is given over the telephone.

Suppliers
Phyto Products Limited Park Works, Park Road, Mansfield Woodhouse, Notts. NG19 8EF. Tel.: 01623 644344.
Manufacturers of a wide range of herbal preparations, including Schoenenberger Cellular Plant Juices. Ring for further information and catalogue.
G. Baldwin & Co. 173 Walworth Road, London SE17 1RW. Tel.: 0171 703 5550.
Suppliers of a large range of herbs, aromatherapy oils, (Solgar stockist) health food store. Worldwide mail order service.
Bioforce (UK) Ltd. Olympic Business Park, Drybridge Road, Dundonald, Ayrshire KA2 9BE. Tel.: 01563 851177.
Neal's Yard Remedies 31 King Street, Manchester M2 6AA. Tel.: 0161 831 7875
Herbal suppliers (mainly Western), wide selection of essential oils, herbal and homoeopathic tinctures and remedies, Bach Flower Remedies. Shop and mail order service.

USA

American Herbalist Guild P.O. Box 746555, Arvada, Colorado 80006.

AUSTRALIA

National Herbalist Association of Australia Suite 14, 247/249 Kingsgrove Road, Kingsgrove, NSW.

HOMOEOPATHY
UK

The Homoeopathic Trust 2 Powis Place, Great Ormond Street, London WC1N 3HT. Tel.: 0171 837 9469.

Organisation governing medically qualified homoeopaths.

The Trust provides an information pack which includes a countrywide list of homoeopathic doctors (both NHS and private). Also details of the NHS referral procedure—either to a local practitioner or homoeopathic hospital.

The Society of Homoeopaths 2 Artizan Road, Northampton NN1 4HU. Tel.: 01604 214000.

Organisation governing non-medically qualified professional homoeopaths. Send A5 sae for their countrywide register of practitioners and information leaflet.

Suppliers

A limited range of remedies can be obtained in health food shops and an increasing number of chemists. Specialist pharmacies and manufacturers supply the full range of homoeopathic remedies. A mail order service is operated by the well-known pharmacies and manufacturers listed below.

Ainsworths Pharmacy 36 New Cavendish Street, London W1M 7LH. Tel.: 0171 935 5330.

Buxton and Grant 176 Whiteladies Road, Bristol BS8 2XU. Tel.: 0117 973 5025.

Freemans of Glasgow Busby Pharmacy, 20 Main Street, Busby, Glasgow G76 8DU. Tel.: 0141 644 1165.

Galen Homoeopathics Lewell Mill, West Stafford, Dorchester, Dorset DT2 8AN. Tel.: 01305 263996 (24-hour message service).

Helios 97 Camden Road, Tunbridge Wells, Kent TN1 2QR. Tel.: 01892 536393/537254 (24-hour message service). Selection of homoeopathic books, stockists of Weleda, Biocare, Solgar, Bach Remedies. Regular talks and pharmacy tours.

A. Nelson & Co. Ltd. 73 Duke Street, Grosvenor Square, London W1M 6BY. Tel.: (0171) 495 2404.

Weleda (UK) Ltd. Heanor Road, Ilkeston, Derbyshire DE7 8DR. Tel.: (0115) 944 8200.

USA

North American Society of Homoeopaths 10700 Old County Road, 15 Suite 33350, Plymouth, Minnesota.

National Centre for Homoeopathy 801 North Fairfax Street, Suite 306, Alexandria, Virginia 22314.

AUSTRALIA

Australian Association of Professional Homoeopaths 80 Essenden Road, Anstead, Queensland 4070.

MACROBIOTICS

Community Health Foundation 188 Old Street, London EC1V 9FR. Tel.: 0171 251 4076.

General information and practitioner details.

Suppliers

Freshlands Health Store 196 Old Street, London EC1V 9FR. Tel.: 0171 250 1708.

Extensive range of macrobiotic foods and cookware, wholefoods, natural healing products, supplements, a variety of organic products, fresh vegetables, fruit, large selection of books. Fresh food takeaway. Therapists available to help with: macrobiotic dietary advice, women's health problems, emotional counselling, healing, homoeopathy, herbal medicine, allergy testing.

USA

Kushi Institute P.O. Box 7, Becket, Massachusetts 01223.

AUSTRALIA

Australian School of Macrobiotics 48 Derwent Street, P.O. Box 705, Glebe 2037.

MEDITATION

School of Meditation 158 Holland Park Avenue, London W11 4UH. Tel.: 0171 603 6116, for general enquiries. The school will also recommend related organisations.

NATURAL PROGESTERONE

UK

Natural Progesterone Information Service P.O. Box 131, Etchingham, East Sussex TN19 7ZN.

Supplies an excellent general information pack, a doctor's information pack, audio tapes, Dr John Lee's books and videos.

Higher Nature Burwash Common, East Sussex TN19 7LX. Tel.: 01435 882 880 (orders only). Nutritionists: 0891 615522.

Source of natural progesterone, other natural hormone products and menopause supplements.

Within the UK, Pro-Gest cream can only be supplied with a doctor's prescription, but the product can be sent by mail order anywhere outside the UK without a prescription. Higher Nature offers qualified nutritionists for telephone consultation and can refer you to a doctor. It also offers a catalogue of herbal and nutritional products and other vitamins and minerals to help the menopause.

IRELAND
The Health Ministry The Nutrition Centre, Donegal Town, County Donegal, Eire. Tel.: 0701 070 3123.
Pro-Gest cream supplied by mail order without prescription. Nutritionist advice available.

NUTRITIONAL THERAPY
Society for the Promotion of Nutritional Therapy P.O. Box 47, Heathfield, East Sussex TN21 8ZX. Tel.: 01435 867007. An educational and campaigning organisation with lay and professional members. Send £1 plus sae for information and a list of therapists in your area.

Suppliers
Nature's Best Health Products P.O. Box 1, Tunbridge Wells, Kent TN2 3EQ. Tel.: 01892 552118.
Mail order catalogue sent upon request. Dietary advisors available.
Solgar Vitamins Ltd. Aldbury, Tring, Herts HP23 5PT. Tel.: 01442 890355.
Telephone for nearest stockist.

Reflexology

Association of Reflexologists 27 Gloucester Street, London WC1N 3XX. Tel./fax: 0990 6733320.

Send A5 sae for countrywide practitioner list, or telephone for name of local practitioner.

GENERAL

Chase Organics Coombelands House, Coombelands Lane, Addlestone, Surrey KT15 1HY. Tel.: 01932 820958.

The Organic Gardening Catalogue. Organic food by mail order.

Greenpeace Canonbury Villas, London N1 2PN. Tel.: 0171 865 8100.

Will provide information on hormone disruptors.

Growing Needs Bookshop 11 Market Place, Glastonbury, Somerset BA6 9HH. Tel.: 01458 833466. Fax: 01458 834040.

Provides an international mail order service.

Helpful Reading

AROMATHERAPY
Aromatherapy, Micheline Arcier, Hamlyn
Aromatherapy, an A–Z, Patricia Davis, C.W. Daniel
Aromatherapy, Christine Westwood, Amberwood

BACH REMEDIES
The Twelve Healers and other Remedies, Edward Bach,
    C.W. Daniel
The Bach Flower Remedies Step by Step, Judy Howard, C.W.
    Daniel
Bach Flower Remedies for Women, Judy Howard, C.W.
    Daniel
Questions and Answers, John Ramsell, C.W. Daniel
The Bach Remedies Repertory, F.J. Wheeler, C.W. Daniel

COUNSELLING
Living Magically, Gill Edwards, Piatkus
Counselling and Helping, Stephen Murgatroyd, The British
    Psychological Society
On Being a Client, David Howe, Sage
The Skilled Healer, Gerard Egan, Brooks/Cole Publishing
    Co.
(Obtainable from Growing Needs Bookshop, Glastonbury,
    Somerset by mail order.)

HEALING
Self Healing, Louis Proto, Piatkus
Spiritual Healing—Energy Medicine for Today, Jack
    Angelo, Element

Spiritual Healing—A Patient's Guide, Eilee Inge Herberg,
    C.W.Daniel

HERBAL MEDICINE
The Herb Society's Complete Medicinal Herbal, Penelope
    Ody, Dorling Kindersley

HOMOEOPATHY
The Complete Guide to Homoeopathy, Dr Andrew Lockie
    and Dr Nicola Geddes, Dorling Kindersley
A Woman's Guide to Homoeopathic Medicine, Dr Trevor
    Smith, Thorsons
Homoeopathy for Women, Rima Handley, Thorsons
Homoeopathy and the Menopause, Beth MacEoin, Thorsons

(HRT) HORMONE REPLACEMENT THERAPY
*Hormone Replacement Therapy - Your Guide to Making
    an Informed Choice*, Rosemary Nicol, Vermillion
Hormone Replacement Therapy, Patsy Westcott, Thorsons

MACROBIOTICS
The Self-Healing Cookbook, Kristina Turner, Earthstone
    Press, California
Food and Healing, Annemarie Colbin, Ballantine Books,
    New York
Healing with Wholefood, Paul Pitchford, North Atlantic
    Books, California

MEDITATION
The Elements of Meditation, David Fontana, Element
The 3 Minute Meditator, David Harp, Piatkus
Trusting the Healer Within, Nick Bamforth, Gateway Books

Creative Visualization, Shakti Gawain, New World Library
Colour Healing, Theo Gimbel, Gaia Books

NATURAL PROGESTERONE
*Natural Progesterone—The Multiple Roles of a
    Remarkable Hormone*, Dr John Lee, John Carpenter
    Publishing
What Your Doctor May Not Tell You About The Menopause,
    Dr John Lee, Warner Books—New York
Both books are available from Higher Nature, the Natural
    Progesterone Information Service and many bookshops)

NUTRITION AND DIET
Principles of Nutritional Therapy, Linda Lazarides, Thorsons
Nutritional Medicine, Dr Stephen Davies and Dr Alan
    Stewart, Pan
You Don't Have to Feel Unwell, Robin Needes, Gateway
The Cranks Recipe Book, Cranks Restaurants, Orion
Rose Elliot's Complete Vegetarian Cookbook, Rose Elliot,
    Harper Collins
The Fit for Life Cookbook Marilyn Diamond, Bantam Books
The Simple Guide to Organic Gardening, Bob Sherman,
    Collins and Brown
The Organics Directory, Clive Litchfield, Green Books

REFLEXOLOGY
Reflexology—A Way to Better Health, Nicola M. Hall,
    Gateway Books
The Reflexology Handbook—A Complete Guide, Laura
    Norman with Thomas Cowan, Piatkus

Relaxation
Stress—How Your Diet Can Help, Stephen Terrass, Thorsons
The Book of Stress Survival, Alix Kirsta, Thorsons
The Stress Protection Plan, Leon Chaitow, Thorsons
Yoga over 50, Mary Stewart, Little, Brown
Stress and Relaxation, Jane Madders, Optima
Managing Stress, Ursula Markham, Element

Shiatsu
Shiatsu for Beginners, Nigel Dawes, Piatkus
Barefoot Shiatsu, Shizuko Yamamoto, Japan Publications
Massage, The Oriental Method, Katsusuke Serizawa, Japan
    Publications
Shiatsu for Women, Ray Ridolfi and Susanne Franzen,
    Thorsons
The Complete Book of Shiatsu Therapy, Toru Namikoshi,
    Japan Publications

Traditional Chinese Medicine
The Complete Illustrated Guide to Chinese Medicine, Tom
    Williams, Element
Traditional Chinese Medicine, Sheila McNamara and Dr
    Song Xuan Ke, Hamish Hamilton

Index